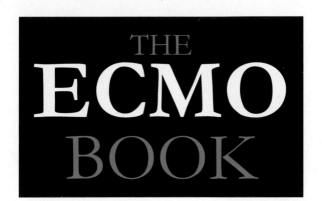

THE
ECMO
BOOK

THE
ECMO
BOOK

Jeffrey DellaVolpe, MD

The Institute for Extracorporeal Life Support

Pulmonary/Sleep Clinic

San Antonio Texas

USA

ELSEVIER

Elsevier
1600 John F. Kennedy Blvd.
Ste 1800
Philadelphia, PA 19103-2899

THE ECMO BOOK

ISBN: 978-0-443-11198-3

Notice

Practitioners and researchers must always rely on their own experience and knowledge in evaluating and using any information, methods, compounds or experiments described herein. Because of rapid advances in the medical sciences, in particular, independent verification of diagnoses and drug dosages should be made. To the fullest extent of the law, no responsibility is assumed by Elsevier, authors, editors or contributors for any injury and/or damage to persons or property as a matter of products liability, negligence or otherwise, or from any use or operation of any methods, products, instructions, or ideas contained in the material herein.

Content Strategist: Michael Houston[†]
Content Development Manager: Ranjana Sharma
Senior Content Development Specialist: Ambika Kapoor
Publishing Services Manager: Shereen Jameel
Project Manager: Maria Shalini
Cover and Design Direction: Amy Buxton
Marketing Manager: Kate Bresnahan

Printed in India.

Last digit is the print number: 9 8 7 6 5 4 3 2

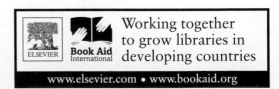

[†] deceased

To the patients and families that have entrusted me with their care in their most vulnerable moments.

ACKNOWLEDGMENTS

If this book proves useful, it is likely due to the experience that I have gained in caring for hundreds and hundreds of patients on ECMO. Gathering this experience is no small feat and stands as a testament to the incredible team that I have in my life.

First and foremost, to my wife Alissa. Your support, love, and dedication means more to me than you know. For the hundreds of times, I had to run out for an emergency, I cannot think of one time that you did not meet me with understanding, even though I know the cost was often great. I am blessed to have you by my side.

To my boys, Luca and Leo, for continuing to remind me of what is important in life and for bringing me a joy that I never knew possible.

To my parents, Dave and Rita, for teaching me that no goal is too large if you have the audacity to set it in your sites, and for showing me the discipline, hard work, and dedication needed to make those goals happen. A special thanks to you Dad, for teaching me how to write.

To my brother and sister, Mark and Mona Lisa, for always being there, and for your friendship, love, and support. I am grateful beyond words to have you in my life.

To the team with the Institute for ECLS, Bradford Anderson, Rachel Sterling, Linda Sousse, Steven Amerson, McKenna Hoffman, and Chris Mathis. Your passion for discovery, innovation, and moving ECMO care forward is a daily inspiration to me. A special thank you to Rachel for reviewing the numerous revisions of this book.

To our team that takes care of all of our patients at the bedside – the nurses, doctors, respiratory therapists, rehabilitation therapists, perfusionists, pharmacists, nutritionists, and case managers. Your tireless and unceasing work is the reason so many patients are now home with their family. The job may seem thankless some days, but know that this is never the case to me. I will forever be grateful for all that you do.

To Jairo Melo and my partners with Texas IPS. Your support on a daily basis to our patients and program means more to me than you will ever know. A special mention to Hitesh Gidwani, Ravi Santhanam, Pavan Thangudu, Shameen Salam, Craig Ainsworth, and Salim Rezaie. If I have slept soundly any night in the last 5 years, it is because I know that you are caring for the patients.

To Chandra Kunavarapu, my partner and brother, for your collaboration, confidence, and the trust that you place in me. It has been an honor building our program together.

To the administrative and leadership team of Methodist Healthcare, especially Dan Miller, Michael John, Allen Harrison, Fernando Triana, and Rachel Goldsmith. Your vision, leadership, and support are the reason our program has been able to save hundreds of lives. You never wavered in your support of me or the program, for which I am forever grateful.

To my mentors who taught me the discipline of critical care – Jason Moore, Ali Al Khafaji, David Huang, and Phil Mason. More than any lesson, you instilled in me a passion for the care of critically ill patients that remains with me to this day.

To the three men who taught me medicine – Andrew Schutzbank, Craig DiTomasso, and Pip Dorsey, for setting the foundation for my entire medical career.

To Father Don Owens, for teaching me to recognize the humanity in every patient I meet – that care of the patient begins with the mind, body, and soul. I am grateful in a special way for your continued friendship to this day.

To Coach Wiese, for teaching me what true dedication to patient care looks like, in lessons spoken and unspoken.

To my colleague, mentor, and friend Tom McRae. It is an honor and a blessing to work alongside you.

Last but not least, a deep debt of gratitude to Brad Johnson, Devin Bowers, Sara Grieshop, Michael Muscat, and Herb Williams-Dalgart. Your passion and tireless advocacy for elevating nursing care to the highest level is palpable, and I count myself fortunate to join the cause in even a small measure.

When I explain ECMO to families of patients, they are skeptical.

"That's it? I thought it was supposed to be complex."

When it comes down to it, the mechanism is deceivingly simple – pumping blood out of the body, allowing oxygen to diffuse in, and returning that blood to the body.

So why is it that providers struggle? Why is it that many ECMO programs fail to apply the support in the right way? And why is it that so many healthcare professionals who manage patients on ECMO struggle to respond in the right way when things go wrong?

This book was written to provide an answer to these questions. ECMO can be both lifesaving and practice changing, but it has to be carried out within the context of a systematic framework for approaching the care of severely decompensated patients in order to be effectively applied at the bedside.

WHAT THIS MATERIAL IS ABOUT

This material proposes a central idea – everything we do for our patients in the ICU comes with a cost. When we add vasopressors, mechanical ventilation, fluids, or medications to our patients' care, we do so to stabilize them and ultimately alter the course of the disease enough to allow for a better outcome. However, all of these interventions come with costs, some subtle and others very overt.

While understanding and quantifying this cost can be well understood in some disciplines of medicine, it is notoriously difficult to quantify the toxicity of care when it comes to critically ill patients because the stakes are so high. We have to accept risk just because of the nature of keeping patients alive can be such a serious proposition.

The effect of the dose-related toxicity of care can not be underestimated. We can increase the dosage of pressors 10-fold over the course of minutes, double or triple the amount of ventilator support due to a desaturation, and apply medications that can affect receptors that are completely undiscovered.

Which leads us to ECMO. If ECMO is applied or even considered as part of a patient's care, it has to be done within the context of toxicity of care. Namely, ECMO must spare some toxicity in order to justify the risks of adding additional support. This is the fundamental principle on which the rest of this book will be built. Once this is established, we will further explore the concepts surrounding ECMO to gradually build a better understanding of this support and how it interacts with the body.

HOW WE WILL DO THIS

Part 1 is going to develop the building blocks and tools that will be used throughout this book. We will start by describing how the body delivers oxygen, the unique characteristics of that mechanism, and, most importantly, how this mechanism breaks down in the setting of severe critical illness. We will then explore the role that critical care interventions have in maintaining oxygen delivery with a focus on the dose-related toxicity that can be associated with high levels of support in severe illness and decompensation.

Part 2 introduces extracorporeal support as a mechanism for sparing this toxicity and describes the clinical scenarios in which it is able to do so. We will discuss selection of patients for ECMO, with special attention to identifying patients in whom ECMO is most likely to benefit and least likely to cause harm. We will also become more familiar with the circuit itself in order to understand the components, alarms, and sensors, in addition to the cannula types and configurations that may be applied.

In Part 3, we are really going to develop our understanding of how extracorporeal support interacts with the body's physiology by taking a deep dive into how this support works. We will explore the dynamics and limits to blood flow, the characteristics of the membrane oxygenator, and the specific ways that ECMO interacts with the body in both respiratory and cardiac support.

Finally, Part 4 will bring it all together, by describing the management principles unique to patients on ECMO. We will build on our framework and principles established in Part 3 and propose how these principles can be applied in day-to-day management in addition to establishing how management can be directed toward sparing toxicity to the maximal extent possible. While the mainstay of management of patients on ECMO is the provision of excellent critical care, our discussion will focus on the points relevant and unique to patients on extracorporeal support.

WHAT THIS MATERIAL IS DESIGNED TO DO

Hopefully at the end of this journey, you will have a much better framework for how the care of patients with severe cardiac and respiratory failure can be managed with extracorporeal support. You will have the tools and principles that can be applied real time to improve the provision of care at the bedside. These principles will not be comprehensive, but can be a framework that you can build upon, adding the knowledge, experience, understanding, and perspective gained from every patient with whose care you are entrusted.

WHAT THIS BOOK IS NOT DESIGNED TO DO

This material is presented humbly, with acknowledgment of what it can provide and what is cannot.

This book is not designed to be comprehensive. On the contrary, it is designed to be succinct, approachable, and understandable, in order to develop a framework that can be built upon. Hopefully this framework can give you a mechanism to apply to specific patient scenarios in order to better contextualize and understand what is happening clinically. There are many approaches to the clinical challenges that you will encounter. To whatever extent possible, specific processes and protocols will be avoided, with the realization that these must be often tailored to the needs of the individual institution and program.

This material is designed to describe the overall principles and experience gathered while taking care of these patients. Therefore, the explanations, illustrations, and concepts are designed to be descriptive rather than definitive.

The material is not to be taken as medical advice. The care of individual patients needs to be put in the context of the specific clinical situation.

And finally, the principles and concepts are primarily developed within the context of the care of adults. While they can certainly be applied to pediatrics in many regards, the majority of the principles have been developed through experience of caring for the adult population.

I look forward to taking this journey together, and am grateful for the opportunity to share the experience, principles, and framework to follow.

CONTENTS

PART I

Physiology

Oxygen Delivery and Consumption

Imagine that you walk into a typical intensive care unit (ICU). You look around and note what you see: in one room a 78-year-old man with urosepsis and septic shock, in the next room a 65-year-old woman with a chronic obstructive pulmonary disease exacerbation, in the next a 55-year-old man with cirrhosis and a gastrointestinal bleed, in the next a 45-year-old man with non-ST-elevation myocardial infarction and intermittent runs of ventricular tachycardia…

The list goes on and on.

What do all of these patients and, frankly, any patient admitted to the ICU have in common? They all have very different pathology, medical histories, and modalities of support that they are requiring.

However, all of these patients are in the ICU because they have a deficiency or are at risk of having a deficiency in their ability to deliver oxygen. This is tremendously important to recognize about our patients – the common reason for critical care interventions is a deficiency in the delivery of oxygen. The better we understand the concept of how oxygen is delivered, the better position we are in to define and support this delivery of oxygen.

HOW IS OXYGEN DELIVERED IN THE BODY?

Have you ever wondered why it is that the tissue that surrounds the heart and lungs is not preferentially oxygenated, compared to the tissue in the periphery (Fig. 1.1)?

At first glance, this is what you might expect. After all, the tissue surrounding the heart and lungs is located centrally and has the nearest proximity to oxygen when it first comes into the body. Indeed, if oxygen was distributed throughout the body by diffusion, then this would be the case.

What do I mean by diffusion? Diffusion is the movement of molecules down their concentration gradient from high concentration to low concentration.

Think of how oxygen enters the body in the lungs – you take a breath in and air enters through your nose/mouth, down your trachea, across your bronchi, all the way to the alveoli. At this point the oxygen *diffuses* into the blood, going from an area of high concentration (the alveoli) to an area of lower concentration (the blood) (Fig. 1.2).

For many organisms such as bacteria, amoebae, and some jellyfish, this process of diffusion is the primary mechanism for the distribution of oxygen. However, all higher levels of function/life are dependent on a more efficient process for oxygen delivery.

Why is diffusion inefficient at delivering oxygen? Let's start by sketching the potential relationship of oxygen delivery by diffusion. If we were to do so, we might expect something that looks like (Fig. 1.3), with a relatively straight line that slopes up, with more delivery of oxygen at higher concentrations and less delivery of oxygen at lower concentrations.

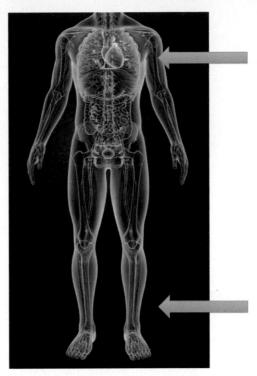

FIG. 1.1 Maintaining oxygenation of both the central and peripheral tissues. (From Sciencepics/Shutterstock.com.)

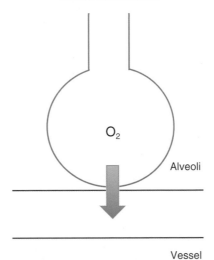

O_2

Alveoli

Vessel

FIG. 1.2 The alveolar-capillary interface as an example of oxygen diffusion in the body

If this were how oxygen were delivered, you would not anticipate much efficiency, as tissues that were present at higher oxygen concentrations (the right side of the line) would have the majority of O_2 delivered and tissues that were present at lower oxygen concentrations (the left side of the line) would have less oxygen delivered. Fortunately, there is a much more efficient means of delivering oxygen.

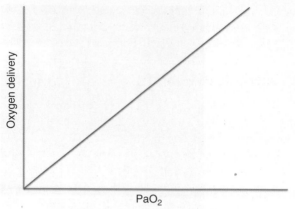

FIG. 1.3 Oxygen delivery by diffusion

WHAT ALLOWS FOR EFFICIENT DELIVERY OF OXYGEN THROUGHOUT THE BODY?

If you were inventing a way to ideally deliver oxygen throughout the body, you would want to have a system that would **bind** preferentially to oxygen, when there is an abundance of oxygen and **dump** preferentially, when there is less presence of oxygen. Returning to our graph, you may ideally expect something like the gray lines below, where there is a lower inflection point, allowing for less delivery/higher binding at high concentrations of oxygen and an upper inflection point, allowing for more delivery/higher dumping at lower concentrations of oxygen (Fig. 1.4).

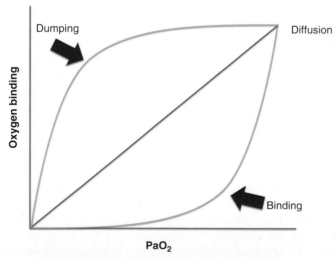

FIG. 1.4 Making oxygen delivery more efficient

Any system that features these two inflection points would be vastly superior and allow for a much more efficient means of delivering oxygen. Fortunately, this is not just an arbitrary thought exercise but, rather, describes the molecule that lies at the center of oxygen delivery – hemoglobin!

HOW DOES HEMOGLOBIN ALLOW FOR MORE EFFICIENT OXYGEN DELIVERY?

Remember the ideal molecule for delivery of oxygen has two properties:
1. Preferentially **bind** when there is an abundance of oxygen

and

2. Preferentially **dump** when there is a scarcity of oxygen

Let's explore how hemoglobin is able to accomplish both of these goals.

Hemoglobin and oxygen binding

Hemoglobin is a dynamic molecule, which carries with it the ability to fold its proteins and change conformation. Its proteins form a bond with oxygen allowing up to four oxygen molecules to bind to each hemoglobin molecule (Fig. 1.5). However, that is only half the story.

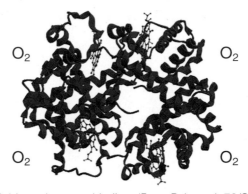

FIG. 1.5 Hemoglobin and oxygen binding. (From Raimundo79/Shutterstock.com.)

Rather than simply binding to oxygen, the hemoglobin molecule carries with it the ability to change its structure based on how much oxygen is bound to it. If a hemoglobin molecule comes into contact with an oxygen molecule, it will bind as noted earlier. However, once it is bound to the first oxygen molecule, hemoglobin changes conformation in such a way that it will bind more strongly to the second O_2 that comes along than the first. Hemoglobin then changes again – the third O_2 is more likely to bind than the second, and the fourth O_2 is more likely to bind than the third.

You can see that this property causes a positive feedback loop, so that as more O_2 comes in contact with more hemoglobin, the amount bound not only increases, but increases in an exponential fashion.

The effect of this is a higher degree of oxygen binding at higher oxygen concentrations (Fig. 1.6).

Hemoglobin and oxygen dumping

Remember, hemoglobin binding in the presence of oxygen abundance is only half the story. The other half is that hemoglobin must also dump oxygen in the periphery, where there is less oxygen available.

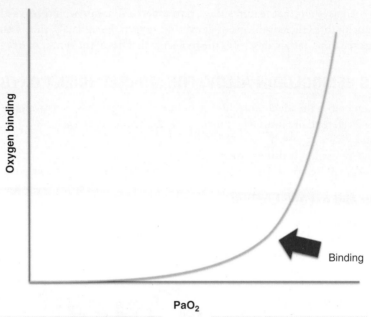

FIG. 1.6 Preferential oxygen binding at high levels of PaO_2

Let's now explore this property of hemoglobin.

The hemoglobin proteins can exist in both a tensed form and a relaxed form. Imagine it as a rubber bowl that can be stretched causing its contents to be spilled out. When hemoglobin exists in the tensed form, oxygen spills out and is dumped for delivery/consumption.

Ideally this tense form would exhibit itself more preferentially in the periphery, which is exactly what happens! This taut form is induced in the presence of higher temperature, lower pH, and higher CO_2 – all conditions common in the periphery (Fig. 1.7A). Thus, each hemoglobin molecule is more likely to be in the tense state and thus dump its oxygen contents in the periphery where there is likely to be less oxygen available (Fig. 1.7B).

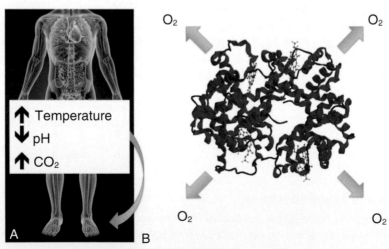

FIG. 1.7 Oxygen conformational changes in periphery. (A, From Sciencepics/Shutterstock.com.; B, From Raimundo79/Shutterstock.com.)

This allow for a system where hemoglobin holds onto oxygen at higher concentrations, only to dump oxygen at lower concentrations (Fig. 1.8).

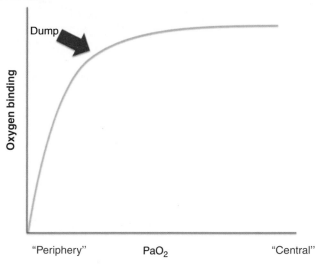

FIG. 1.8 Preferential oxygen dumping at periphery

Taken together, we have the properties of both the lower and the upper inflection points as illustrated below in Fig. 1.9.

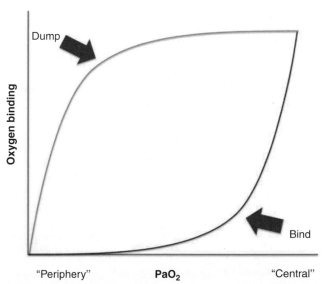

FIG. 1.9 The dual function of hemoglobin - central binding and peripheral dumping

When taken together, these lower and upper inflection points manifest themselves as the sigmoid shape, which is observed in the relationship of hemoglobin binding to oxygen concentration, otherwise known as the hemoglobin dissociation curve (Fig. 1.10).

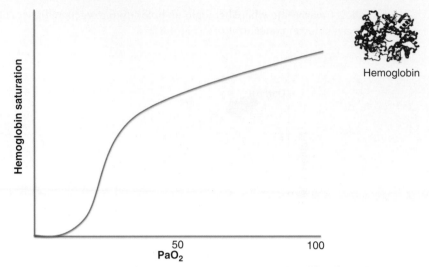

FIG. 1.10 The oxygen hemoglobin dissociation curve. (Modified from Raimundo79/Shutterstock.com.)

Since hemoglobin has the ability to change its conformation, this curve has the ability to shift based on the conditions present. Higher CO_2, lower pH, and higher temperature cause this curve to shift to the right, meaning that in the heart/lungs, hemoglobin is more likely to bind, while in the periphery, it is more likely to dump (Fig. 1.11).

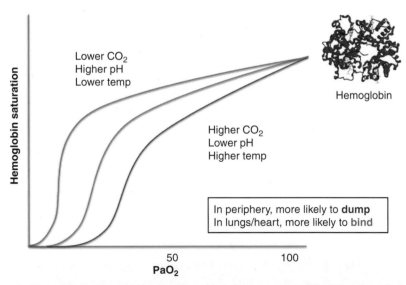

FIG. 1.11 Shifting of the hemoglobin oxygen dissociation curve. (Modified from Raimundo79/Shutterstock.com.)

WHAT IS THE SIGNIFICANCE OF ALL OF THIS WHEN IT COMES TO DELIVERY OF OXYGEN?

This is all so important because the result is that oxygen can be delivered more efficiently. How much more efficiently? Seventy to eighty times more efficient!

Let me say that again, because I think it is the essential point. Because of the efficiency of the hemoglobin molecule, oxygen can be delivered with 70–80 times more efficiently than if by diffusion alone.

Besides instilling a new healthy respect for what hemoglobin is able to do, it also says something about oxygen delivery – the more we can leverage this efficiency, the better we can optimize oxygen delivery, especially when we are in a compromised state.

The new paradigm – oxygen delivery

Understanding oxygen delivery is the ultimate responsibility of anyone taking care of a patient in a critical care setting. The better we can understand, quantify, and optimize the delivery of oxygen, the more equipped we will be for taking care of our patients, even if they are the most compromised patients in the hospital.

How is oxygen delivery defined?

The temptation is that if we want to provide more oxygen delivery, we just provide more oxygen right? Just crank up the O_2 on the wall and we are all set? Wrong! Remember, we have a molecule at our disposal that is 70–80x more efficient than if we were to just rely on diffusion alone. So how do we leverage the efficiency of hemoglobin?

Let's use a common analogy to illustrate this point.

If you have to transport boxes of goods from point A to point B, and you have a truck that is the most efficient carrier of these goods, what are the ways that you can optimize the delivery of these boxes? We should be able to quickly reason that there are only three ways of doing this (Fig. 1.12A):

1. Maximize the load on these trucks.
2. Put more trucks on the road.
3. Have the trucks drive faster.

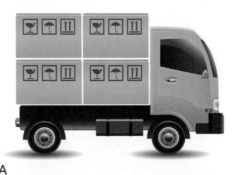

A

FIG. 1.12A The role of hemoglobin in oxygen delivery. (A, From Bannosuke/Shutterstock.com.)

Let's now extend this analogy to think about oxygen. Now, instead of boxes of goods, let's substitute oxygen, such that the parameters become (Fig. 1.12B):

1. Maximally load up these trucks→increase oxygen saturation.
2. Put more trucks on the road→increase hemoglobin.
3. Have the trucks drive faster→increase cardiac output.

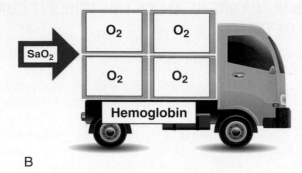

B

FIG. 1.12B The role of hemoglobin in oxygen delivery. (B, From Bannosuke/Shutterstock.com.)

These variables are the basis of the delivery of oxygen equation, which can be written out as:

$$DO_2 = 1.34 \times SaO_2 \times Hb \times CO + PaO_2 \times 0.003$$

How does this apply for your patient?

Let's say you walk into your ICU and see two different patients, Patient A and Patient B. Actually, you see Patient B, but you are *shown* Patient A.

That is because everyone is flagging you to look at Patient A. The respiratory therapist wants you to look at the blood gas that was just drawn, where the PaO_2 is marked as severely abnormal. The bedside nurse is nervously showing you her calculations of cardiac output, which is only calculated to be 6 L per minute.

Patient B meanwhile is off to the side, with few people concerned about his clinical data. The data of Patients A and B are as follows:

Patient A: PaO_2 40 mmHg, Hb 15 g/dL, CO 6 L
Patient B: PaO_2 100 mmHg, Hb 7.5 g/dL, CO 8 L

Knowing what you know now, which patient is more efficiently delivering oxygen?

By doing some simple math, you can see that Patient A is actually delivering more oxygen than Patient B. This is because in this example his hemoglobin concentration is twice as high, allowing him to leverage the efficiency of hemoglobin to a higher degree (Fig. 1.13).

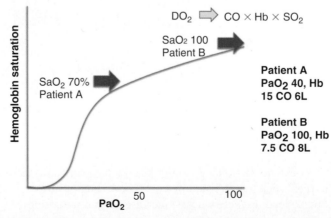

FIG. 1.13 Delivery of oxygen based on different clinical characteristics

HOW IS PAO$_2$ DIFFERENT FROM SAO$_2$?

Let's differentiate between SaO$_2$ (oxygen saturation of hemoglobin) and PaO$_2$ (concentration of oxygen in the blood). Both are often used as a surrogate for how well we are oxygenating, so much so that they are often interchangeable. But you can quickly start to see how different they are!

PaO$_2$ refers to that partial pressure of oxygen, the dissolved amount of oxygen in the blood. SaO$_2$ refers to the overall saturation of hemoglobin. While it is true that higher PaO$_2$ will correspond to a higher hemoglobin O$_2$ saturation (think of the oxygen-hemoglobin dissociation curve) you can see why they are very different, when it comes to what matters the most to the cells of the body – the delivery of oxygen!

The PaO$_2$ of the blood in and of itself only allows for delivery of oxygen via diffusion– a much less efficient process. Which is why its contribution to DO$_2$ is multiplied by a modifier of 0.03 in the DO$_2$ equation.

Doesn't PaO$_2$ just correspond to how saturated the hemoglobin molecule is, and therefore the PaO$_2$?

Are you justified in increasing the FiO$_2$ whenever the blood gas machine flags an abnormal PaO$_2$? Maybe, maybe not.

Remember, the curve shifts depending on what is going on with your patient (Fig. 1.14).

A curve that is shifted to the left (as illustrated by the *green curve*) has a corresponding hemoglobin saturation that is much higher than a curve that is shifted to the right (the *red curve*). And as we will shortly see, in oxygen delivery as in life, there is a cost for every increase in support that we provide.

What ultimately matters to your patient is the DO$_2$. No exceptions!

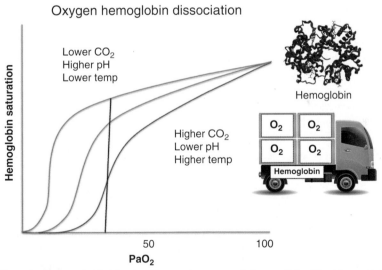

FIG. 1.14 Oxygen hemoglobin dissocation and oxygen delivery. (Modified from Raimundo79/ Shutterstock.com, Bannosuke/Shutterstock.com.)

THE ROLE OF OXYGEN CONSUMPTION

Ok, maybe with one exception.

The other side of the delivery of oxygen is the consumption of oxygen. While oxygen delivery is paramount, it must always be put into the context of consumption. Oxygen delivery is only as good as it relates to the body's consumption needs (Fig. 1.15).

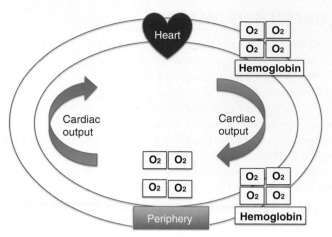

FIG. 1.15 Effect of oxygen consumption in the periphery

To better illustrate this concept, let's imagine ourselves on a treadmill. We are standing on a treadmill at the beginning of our workout. Assuming no deficiencies in our body's ability to deliver oxygen, we are on top of the world, we can stand there indefinitely and feel comfortable that our body is meeting all of its consumption needs.

Now let's start the treadmill and slowly start to increase the speed. What happens? As the treadmill clicks up, from level 1 to 5 to 10, we notice some changes, subtle at first but then becoming more pronounced. Maybe at first we notice that our heart rate is increasing, we start breathing faster, we go from having a full on conversation with the person working out next to us, to speaking in shortened sentences. As the intensity of the treadmill increases higher and higher, we may even start to feel physical pain, distress, our vision blurring, the feeling of oncoming collapse. What is happening here?

What is intuitively happening is that our body is adjusting to match up our DO_2 to our consumption needs, otherwise known as VO_2.

What does this relationship look like?

If we were to plot the relationship of DO_2 and VO_2 it would look something like this, with every increase in VO_2 (as represented by our increasing levels on the treadmill), represented by progressively higher curves (A to B to C) (Fig. 1.16)

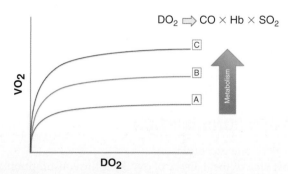

FIG. 1.16 Delivery versus consumption of oxygen at higher levels of consumption

The relationship between DO_2 and VO_2 works in our favor, in that there is a significant amount of redundancy and ability to increase as needed (like we are discovering on our theoretical treadmill). This ability to augment DO_2 (represented by the flat portion of the curve) can readily be increased by 5–6× just by increasing our cardiac output. This is what is happening as our treadmill level is increased, and we experience our heart rate increase.

The other redundancy that is built into this relationship is that body only consumes a fraction of the overall oxygen delivered. How can we know and quantify how much we are consuming? Let's explore.

Quantifying VO_2

VO_2 can be difficult to measure directly; therefore we can infer the overall consumption by comparing how much oxygen is being delivered and how much is being returned to the heart. We can envision that as blood is circulated around the body through the periphery, there will be some oxygen that is used and some that is not. The higher the saturation of blood that returns to the heart, the higher the ratio of DO_2 to VO_2 is, as shown in Fig. 1.17.

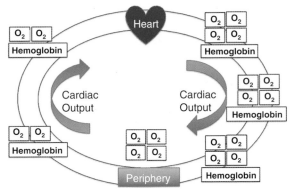

FIG. 1.17 Measuring VO_2

A normal DO_2:VO_2 ratio might be somewhere between 4:1 and 5:1. This means that we are at any point delivering 4 to 5 times the oxygen as the body needs to consume. This is helpful and allows us to continue to increase our overall VO_2 without the collapse that would be expected at the falloff on the left side of the graph (Fig. 1.18).

However, as we increase the VO_2 from point A to point B, you can observe that the delivery of oxygen has to increase in order to continue to maintain the same DO_2:VO_2 ratio. If this is not done, the ratio of DO_2:VO_2 falls from 5:1 to 4:1 or from 4:1 to 3:1 (Fig. 1.18).

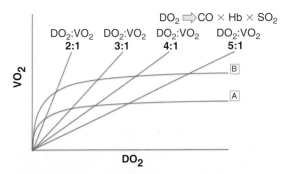

FIG. 1.18 Delivery versus consumption of oxygen

How do we observe this? We can look at the saturation of blood returning to the heart in the form of the venous oxygen saturation. As the DO_2:VO_2 ratio falls from 5:1 to 4:1, the body then has to consume a higher percentage of the total oxygen delivered, and you would expect the venous oxygen saturation to fall from 80% to 75%. This continues until the DO_2:VO_2 ratio falls to 2:1, where you might expect the venous oxygen saturation to perhaps fall to 50%. Which, as you can observe on our graph, is coming closer and closer to the falloff point of the graph and overall collapse.

It is this collapse that we are attempting to prevent in every patient admitted to the ICU.

We will now spend the next several chapters understanding how this collapse occurs and what we can do to stop it.

SUGGESTED READING

Gattinoni, L., Brazzi, L., Pelosi, P., Latini, R., Tognoni, G., & Pesenti, A., et al. (1995). A trial of goal-oriented hemodynamic therapy in critically ill patients. *New England Journal of Medicine, 333*(16), 1025–1032.

Hamilton, C., Steinlechner, B., Gruber, E., Simon, P., & Wollenek, G. (2004). The oxygen dissociation curve: quantifying the shift. *Perfusion, 19*(3), 141–144.

Jensen, F. B. (2009). The dual roles of red blood cells in tissue oxygen delivery: oxygen carriers and regulators of local blood flow. *Journal of Experimental Biology, 212*(21), 3387–3393.

Kruse, J. A., Haupt, M. T., Puri, V. K., & Carlson, R. W. (1990). Lactate levels as predictors of the relationship between oxygen delivery and consumption in ARDS. *Chest, 98*(4), 959–962.

Ranney, H., & Sharma, V. (2000). Structure and function of hemoglobin. *Willimas hematology* (6th ed., pp. 345–353). McGraw Hill.

2

Shock

What is meant by shock? Let's return to our two intensive care unit (ICU) patients.

Patient A: BP 100/40, HR 114, UOP < 10 mL

Patient B: BP 80/40, HR 85, UOP 50 mL/hr

Which patient is in shock? Patient A? Patient B? Both?

WHAT IS SHOCK?

Often the bias is to define shock simply as a low blood pressure. While this is certainly part of the equation, it is not the whole picture.

Why is low blood pressure usually the first thing we think about when we think about shock? Usually, it is because this is the first parameter that presents itself – the monitor starts beeping, alarms are going off, and people around us start getting concerned. However, we have to remember that a low blood pressure, specifically a low mean arterial pressure (MAP), may or may not mean that a patient is in shock (Fig. 2.1).

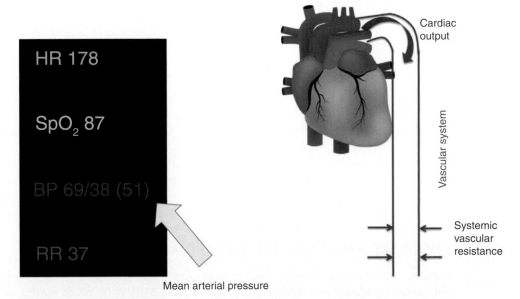

FIG. 2.1 Shock: blood pressure versus cardiac output. (Modified from Ody_Stocker/Shutterstock.com.)

WHAT IS THE DIFFERENCE BETWEEN LOW BLOOD PRESSURE AND SHOCK?

Shock is defined as circulatory failure causing inadequate delivery of oxygen to meet oxygen consumption requirements, leading to cellular and tissue hypoxia. It all comes back to $DO_2:VO_2$. When DO_2 is not adequate to keep up with VO_2, shock ensues.

This is an important distinction from blood pressure. A low MAP can be evidence of a low cardiac output and, thus, a deficiency of $DO_2:VO_2$, but it does not mean that the patient is in shock.

Rather, the MAP is an observed value calculated by the systolic and diastolic blood pressure, which is ultimately a factor of cardiac output, central venous pressure (CVP) to a lesser degree, and systemic vascular resistance (SVR) (Fig. 2.2).

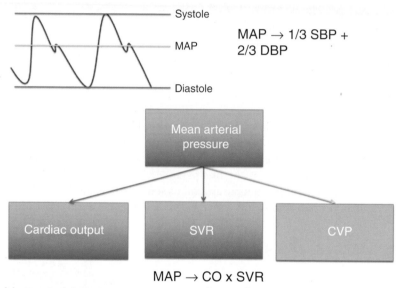

FIG. 2.2 Mean arterial pressure as a surrogate for cardiac output. *CVP*, Central venous pressure; *SVR*, systemic vascular resistance.

We are making this distinction because, ultimately, it does not matter to end organs what the MAP is, but rather how much oxygen is being delivered. It is tempting to chase after specific MAP targets, but these targets only matter to the degree that they are an observed manifestation of cardiac output and ultimately DO_2.

If you measured the blood pressure of 100 random people, you would notice that there is a vast difference in the overall MAP. Some would have a very high MAP and some may have a very low MAP. The people with the lower MAP likely are not in shock. They may have completely adequate perfusion, normal lacatate levels, great urine output, and overall, adequate DO_2.

WHAT IS THE RELATIONSHIP OF MAP TO CARDIAC OUTPUT?

There are certainly some people who if you measured their MAP throughout the course of their normal day (especially during sleep), you might notice a MAP of 65, 60, 55 mmHg, or even below. What is going on with these people? Are we catching shock that would normally go unrecognized?

Clearly not. What we are uncovering here is that MAP only relates to low oxygen delivery to the degree that it is an observable indicator of cardiac output. The reason why some people can maintain adequate oxygen delivery and cardiac output at a lower MAP is SVR.

SVR represents the overall tone of the blood vessels. The normal relation of MAP to SVR is traditionally expressed as:

$$MAP \rightarrow CO \times SVR$$

Thus, we can imagine that the same cardiac output, as represented by the green line, could correspond to very different MAPs, based on what the overall SVR is, as illustrated in Fig. 2.3.

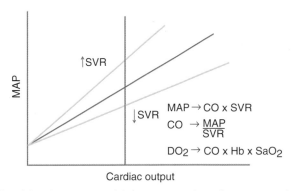

FIG. 2.3 The relationship of mean arterial pressure and cardiac output: the role of systemic vascular resistance. *MAP*, Mean arterial pressure; *SVR*, systemic vascular resistance.

Rather than stating that MAP is a function of CO and SVR, we can consider reframing the relationship as:

$$CO \rightarrow \frac{MAP}{SVR}$$

In this regard, we can see that MAP is the observable manifestation of cardiac output as a function of SVR maintained by the blood vessels. SVR is a derived value and MAP is a measured value. Ultimately, both help to describe the cardiac output and, ultimately, the DO_2.

REFRAMING HOW WE DEFINE SHOCK

Let's return to our DO_2:VO_2 relationship. Remember that as DO_2:VO_2 decreases to below 2:1, we begin to head toward cardiopulmonary and total system collapse (Fig. 2.4).

In order to determine how oxygen is being delivered, we must recognize inadequate delivery of oxygen above all else. If a patient has a normal blood pressure because the SVR is high but oxygen is not being delivered, he or she may be in shock. If a different patient has lower blood pressure because of a lower SVR, but oxygen is being delivered, urine output is adequate, mental status is maintained, and all tissues have evidence of adequate perfusion, shock may not be present, regardless of what the blood pressure is.

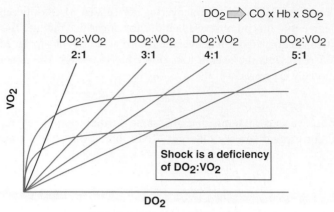

FIG. 2.4 Shock and DO_2:VO_2

HOW DO WE CLASSIFY SHOCK?

Now that we have the framework to recognize shock as a deficiency of oxygen delivery, let's turn our attention to identifying the cause of shock. You will come to appreciate this as the essential piece to managing a patient in shock. Once you know what you are up against, you will be in a much better position to intervene and improve the outcome for your patient.

The traditional classification of shock is based on the relative contributions of low cardiac output and SVR: cardiogenic, obstructive, hypovolemic, and distributive (Fig. 2.5).

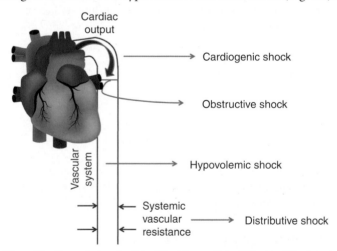

FIG. 2.5 Classification of shock. (Modified from Ody_Stocker/Shutterstock.com.)

It is often tempting to think of these as fixed classifications, with each patient being assigned a designation when they hit the ICU just as they are assigned a medical record number. Your patient with NSTEMI? Cardiogenic shock. Your patient with urosepsis? Distributive shock.

Unfortunately, it is never this simple – each classification can have a multitude of mechanisms, pathophysiologic processes, and etiologies associated. Pericardial tamponade, pulmonary embolism, and pneumothorax can all cause obstructive shock but obstruct in very different ways. The distributive shock caused by anaphylaxis is very different from distributive shock due to sedation effect or neurogenic shock. Even distributive shock due to sepsis can be very different both clinically and on the cellular level when caused by different pathogens (Fig. 2.6).

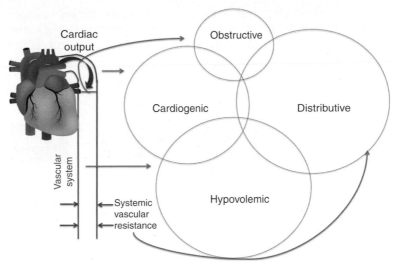

FIG. 2.6 Shock as a clinical spectrum. (Modified from Ody_Stocker/Shutterstock.com.)

These etiologies can often run together, where components of multiple types of shock can be exhibited for a single patient at different points in the clinical course.

Ultimately, classifications are only as useful as their ability to help understand the physiology specific to the patient.

UNCOVERING THE TRUE ETIOLOGY OF SHOCK

The example of distributive shock can be telling. Often when distributive shock is diagnosed, we correctly identify a dysregulation of SVR. However, it is often tempting to think of vascular resistance as the homogenous capability of the blood vessels to provide vascular tone.

However, this lack of tone may be complex in its etiology. Vascular tone is maintained by a vascular endothelium and vascular smooth muscle, with a variety of hormones, neurotransmitters, and vasoactive factors maintaining the endothelium and a host of receptors and cofactors affecting the vascular smooth muscle (Fig. 2.7).

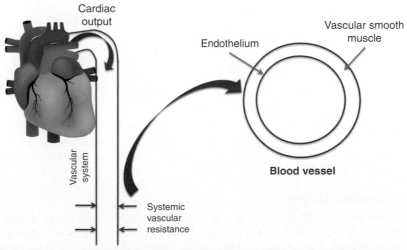

FIG. 2.7 The components of vascular tone. (Modified from Ody_Stocker/Shutterstock.com.)

This complex system allows for patients to differ not only in their presentation, but their response to therapy. A patient whose loss of vascular tone is primarily a function of decreased stimulation by the adrenergic nervous system may respond particularly well to epinephrine, while a patient whose tone is primarily due to a relative deficiency in antidiuretic hormone may respond much better to vasopressin.

In reality there are a host of deficiencies that can be responsible for this loss of vascular tone, which are illustrated in Fig. 2.8.

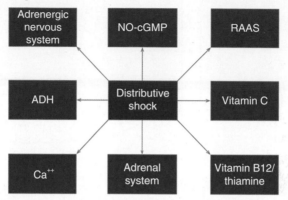

FIG. 2.8 The multiple components required to maintain vascular tone. *ADH*, Antidiuretic hormone; *NO-cGMP*, nitric oxide cyclic guanosine monophosphate; *RAAS*, renin-angiotensin-aldosterone system.

We often note the effect clinically – that our patient "responded really well to vasopressin" or "really liked the calcium." Overall, this serves to remind us that shock can be complex in its etiology, and that the classifications that we set up are designed to better understand the physiology that is unique to the patient.

OPTIMIZING CARDIAC OUTPUT IN SHOCK

So what do we do about shock? How can we improve our cardiac output? The traditional consideration is to put it into the context of preload, afterload, and contractility (Fig. 2.9).

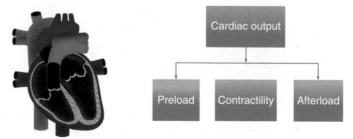

FIG. 2.9 Cardiac output and the contribution of preload, afterload, and contractility. (Modified from Ody_Stocker/Shutterstock.com.)

Let's discuss the individual components.

Preload and cardiac output

When considering preload, consider a slingshot. If you were to load a pebble on a slingshot and draw back the band, the pebble would fly a certain distance. Now, let's envision pulling the band back further … the pebble will fly further. Draw back further still, and the pebble will fly further.

However, you can also envision that as we continue to draw back further and further, the distance the pebble will fly begins to become less and less. After a certain point, we experience progressively diminishing returns for further increases. In fact, if we were to plot this relationship on a graph, you might expect something as follows, where there is higher responsiveness to preload initially, followed by less responsiveness with progressive increases in preload (Fig. 2.10).

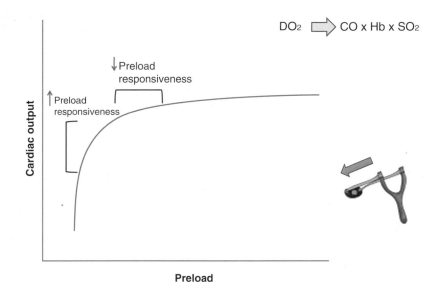

FIG. 2.10 Cardiac output as a function of preload. (Modified from Pashigorov/PREMIUM Stock Vector/Shutterstock.)

This relationship is what we observe with regard to preload and cardiac output. There is a point where preload corresponds to a significant increase in cardiac output, and a point where there is less responsiveness of cardiac output to preload.

What is the effect of afterload?

Conversely, let's consider the effect of afterload. In this case, envision the effect of pushing a box across the room. Now, imagine adding weight to the box to make it progressively heavier. Initially, the heavier box barely impacts your ability to push the box across the room. However, at a certain point, there will be a rapid decline in the ability to push this box.

Just like different people are able to push different size boxes, the response to afterload can be varied based on the capabilities of the heart. Regardless of the overall tolerance to afterload, the pattern is a period of minimal effects of afterload, followed by a sharp decline in cardiac output (Fig. 2.11).

Preload and afterload in the setting of the right and left heart

Although this convention of preload and afterload is often applied to the heart as a whole, it can sometimes be helpful to think of the effect of preload and afterload as they relate to the left and right heart.

Specifically, the right heart offers the opportunity to consider the effect of preload and afterload in a unique way, which may help to explain the clinical characteristics that we observe at the bedside (Fig. 2.12).

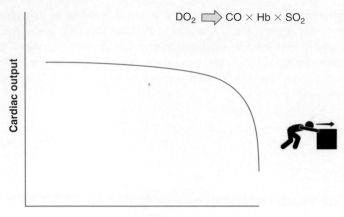

$$DO_2 \implies CO \times Hb \times SO_2$$

FIG. 2.11 Cardiac output as a function of afterload. (Modified from Leremy/Stock Illustrations/ Shutterstock.)

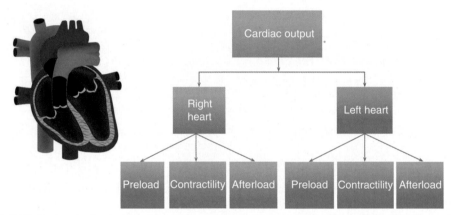

FIG. 2.12 Preload, afterload, and contractility of the left and right heart. (Modified from Ody_ Stocker/Shutterstock.com.)

The right heart behaves very differently from the left heart. Where the left heart is designed to push blood through the entire systemic circulation, the right heart is primarily designed to pump blood through the pulmonary circulation. This difference in function is reflected in differences in form – in general, it is less muscular, contracts on a different axis, and exhibits different responses to filling pressures.

Being less muscular, the right heart exhibits a less robust response to preload with an abrupt stop due to limitations of the pericardium. The effect of preload on the left and right heart is illustrated in Fig. 2.13.

This means that there is a limit to how much volume can be administered to augment the right heart output. At a certain point, the stretch afforded by additional volume only translates into more dilation of the right ventricular cavity, which can have an adverse effect on cardiac output.

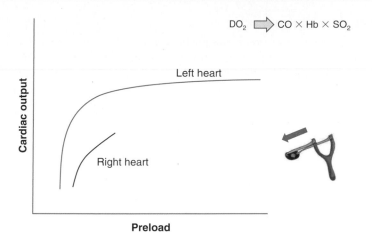

FIG. 2.13 Preload effect for the left and right heart. (Modified from Pashigorov/PREMIUM Stock Vector/Shutterstock.)

How does excess preload adversely affect cardiac output in a failing right ventricle?

When preload is given to a right ventricle that is no longer preload responsive, the right ventricle can only expand across the septum, which in turn compresses the left ventricle (Fig. 2.14).

Doing so may actually drop the left ventricular preload, which can be observed clinically – when fluid is administered in the setting of right ventricular failure, the blood pressure may actually go down.

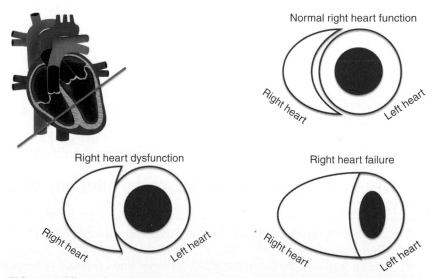

FIG. 2.14 Effect of preload on failing right ventricle. (Modified from Ody_Stocker/Shutterstock.com.)

Afterload and the right ventricle

In a similar manner to the unique effects of preload on the right ventricle, afterload can have a profound impact on the overall function of the right ventricle. Being less muscular and contracting on a different axis, the right ventricle is exquisitely sensitive to the effects of afterload, with a sharp drop-off in function with even modest increases in afterload (Fig. 2.15).

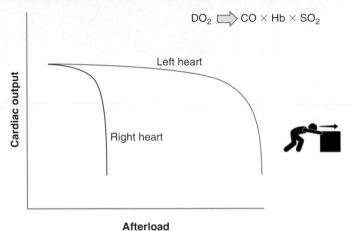

$$DO_2 \Rightarrow CO \times Hb \times SO_2$$

FIG. 2.15 Cardiac output as a function of afterload for the left and right heart. (Modified from Leremy/Stock Illustrations /Shutterstock.)

Variables increasing right ventricular afterload

Since the right ventricle is pumping through the pulmonary circulation, anything that increases pulmonary vascular resistance (PVR) increases this afterload and carries with it the risk of worsening right ventricular output.

Can this happen for conditions that are commonly encountered in the ICU? Absolutely! Let's review some of the factors that increase PVR, which certainly are recognizable for many patients you may encounter in the ICU:
1. Hypercapnia (elevated CO_2)
2. Hypoxia
3. Acidosis
4. Hypothermia
5. Decreased lung compliance (from pneumonia, edema, atelectasis, etc.)
6. Elevated adrenergic tone

You can quickly envision the many situations that you might encounter in the ICU where right ventricular afterload can escalate and you can observe a rapid decline in right heart function.

HOW CAN WE USE THIS MODEL OF SHOCK TO IMPROVE THE MANAGEMENT OF OUR PATIENTS?

Models are only helpful in the way they help us to approach and think about what we are observing clinically.

Let's say you see a patient in the ICU with a low blood pressure. What is our approach to this patient?

First, let's evaluate the patient. Is this blood pressure allowing for adequate delivery of oxygen? Are they making adequate urine? Are they awake and talking? Are they warm and well perfused? Are there lab abnormalities?

If they are in shock, the question becomes what is the shock caused by? Are their clinical and historical data pointing to cardiogenic? Distributive? Obstructive? Or is this perhaps a mixed picture with components of more than one type?

Now we are faced with what do we do about shock. Let's address the role of two of the most common interventions in the ICU for shock – intravenous fluid and vasopressor administration.

Rationale for fluid administration in shock

The entire aim of the administration of fluid in shock is to increase preload to the left ventricle and thus increase cardiac output. But let's think through what this scenario looks like and what assumptions must be true for this to occur.

Even though the intended effect is left ventricular output, we are administering fluid to the venous side of the circulation. The following assumptions must be true for this to translate to an increase in left ventricular output:

1. Enough fluid must stay in the intravascular space to increase right ventricular preload.
2. The preload must increase the right ventricular output.
3. The increase in right ventricular output must be significant enough to augment left ventricular preload.
4. The left ventricle responsive to preload.

Often these assumptions are all true; however, if they are not, then the effect of this additional volume only increases the hydrostatic pressure in the venous system, causing the buildup of fluid in the interstitium and edema (Fig. 2.16).

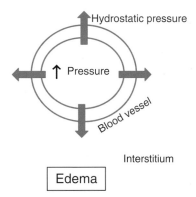

FIG. 2.16 Increased hydrostatic pressure and formation of tissue edema

What is the clinical effect of this edema? Sometimes it is trivial, but for the majority of tissues and organ systems (brain, lungs, heart gut, liver, kidneys, etc.), edema worsens the overall function.

Does this mean that fluids should not be administered in shock? Certainly not! Rather, the point of this exercise is to highlight that our goal should be to optimize DO_2. The way fluids are able to accomplish this is through optimization of cardiac output by increasing preload. Administration of fluid for the mitigation of shock should be done in this context, and we should always assess the response to fluids for evidence that an improvement in oxygen delivery has occurred.

How can pressors help in shock?

For the patient in shock who is unresponsive to fluids, the next step is often to consider the use of vasopressors. The reasoning is sound – if there is a vasodilatory component of shock, vasopressors can improve vascular tone, increasing SVR and, therefore, the blood pressure.

Does this help to mitigate shock? Remember that shock is harmful to the degree that it impairs the ability to deliver oxygen sufficient for the body's needs. Increasing the MAP by increasing SVR does not necessarily translate into an improved DO_2.

Instead, we have to remember that increasing SVR can help to optimize DO_2 by improving vascular tone, and ultimately optimizing venous return and cardiac output. If we are not achieving this, we will see an improvement in MAP but not necessarily an improvement in the delivery of oxygen.

How can we know we are improving cardiac output with our interventions and not just increasing our blood pressure? The answer lies in the physiologic response. For every intervention that we perform, we should ask ourselves "is the intervention that I just performed helping the patient in some meaningful way?" We should ask ourselves if there is an improvement in urine output, a decrease in lactic acid level, or an improvement in liver function tests. Evaluation of the patient before and after an intervention can provide powerful insight into what is going on and can help to guide what interventions are appropriate.

So which pressor should I use?

Hopefully by now, it should be apparent that shock is a complex phenomenon, with a variety of etiologies, manifestations, and physiologic phenomena. It could be classified as primarily cardiogenic, distributive, obstructive, or hypovolemic and could have very different responses to therapy.

To better clarify the effect of pressors in shock, we should understand the effect they have on the cardiac contractility, the systemic vasculature, and importantly on the pulmonary vasculature, which will be critical in the case of any right ventricular failure.

What will follow is not a comprehensive overview but, rather a framework that can be used to approach some of the most common pressors/inotropes utilized when managing a patient in shock.

Norepinephrine

Norepinephrine is one of the most common pressors used. It provides vasoconstriction as well as some inotropy at higher doses, as denoted by the *green arrows*. In this regard, it can be a very useful pressor.

However, note that it can increase the PVR, denoted by the *red arrow*. In patients with a struggling right ventricle, with evidence of right ventricular failure, or at risk for having elevated PVR (hypoxia, acidosis, hypercarbia, etc.) it may worsen the overall right ventricular afterload (Fig. 2.17).

Additionally, like all pressors, it works by stimulation of the adrenergic system. In patients who are in shock due to other reasons, up-titration of this pressor or any pressor may increase the risk of harm with providing minimal benefit.

Epinephrine

Epinephrine is like norepinephrine, with vasoconstrictor and inotropic effects. It can have more of an effect on inotropy with minimal effects on PVR, making it a potential option in patients with right ventricular failure (Fig. 2.18).

Dopamine

Dopamine is dose responsive, which can cause inotropy/chronotropy with the addition of vasoconstriction at higher doses. The higher doses can be associated with higher incidence of arrhythmias, so caution should be made with titration of dopamine (and all vasoactive medications) at higher doses (Fig. 2.19).

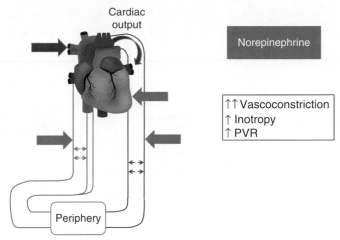

FIG. 2.17 Effects of norepinephrine on cardiac output. *PVR*, Pulmonary vascular resistance. (Modified from Ody_Stocker/Shutterstock.com.)

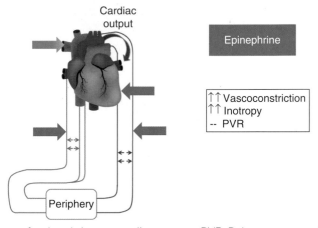

FIG. 2.18 Effects of epinephrine on cardiac output. *PVR*, Pulmonary vascular resistance. (Modified from Ody_Stocker/Shutterstock.com.)

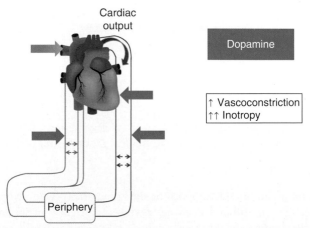

FIG. 2.19 Effects of dopamine on cardiac output. (Modified from Ody_Stocker/Shutterstock.com.)

Vasopressin

Vasopressin is a pure vasopressor. It has no cardiac activity. The increase in cardiac output that ensues is due to improved SVR and improved ventricular preload.

Importantly, as opposed to norepinephrine, vasopressin has minimal effect on PVR (Fig. 2.20).

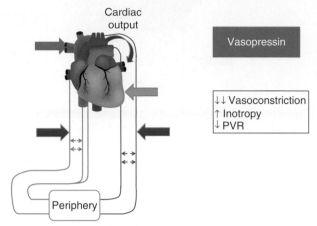

FIG. 2.20 Effects of vasopressin on cardiac output. *PVR*, Pulmonary vascular resistance. (Modified from Ody_Stocker/Shutterstock.com.)

Phenylephrine

Phenylephrine is another pure vasoconstrictor. At higher doses, it can worsen both left and right ventricular afterload and can have the effect of dropping cardiac output. Attention to worsening evidence of shock should be paid to monitor for these effects (Fig. 2.21).

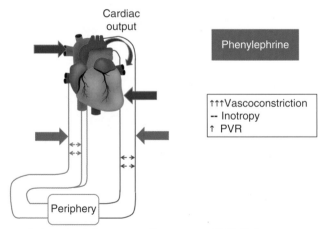

FIG. 2.21 Effects of phenylephrine on cardiac output. *PVR*, Pulmonary vascular resistance (Modified from Ody_Stocker/Shutterstock.com.)

Dobutamine

Dobutamine can provide support for shock in patients who primarily need more inotropy. It can be particularly useful in the setting of worsening right ventricular failure. At higher doses, it can cause vasodilation, so the dose-response relationship should be carefully monitored. It can be initiated at a fixed dose in order to better monitor for these effects (Fig. 2.22).

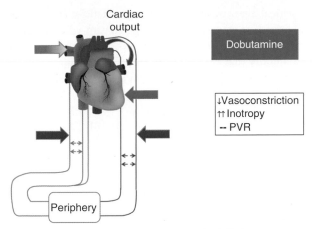

FIG. 2.22 Effects of dobutamine on cardiac output. *PVR*, Pulmonary vascular resistance. (Modified from Ody_Stocker/Shutterstock.com.)

Milrinone

Milrinone is an inotrope that increases cardiac blood flow, reduces afterload, and reduces PVR. This can have the effect of augmenting cardiac output and improving shock. The adverse effect is that it can worsen peripheral vasodilation, thus causing worsening hypotension in patients who have a distributive component to their shock (Fig. 2.23).

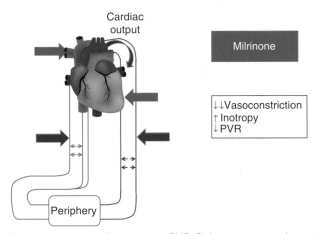

FIG. 2.23 Effects of milrinone on cardiac output. *PVR*, Pulmonary vascular resistance. (Modified from Ody_Stocker/Shutterstock.com.)

PUTTING IT TOGETHER

Anyone who has taken care of critically ill patients has likely seen the devastating effects of shock. The failure to adequately provide oxygen to the end organs can lead to decompensation and death in a rapid and overwhelming fashion.

Understanding shock and the shock state can be complex, and this chapter is by no means comprehensive. However, we hopefully were able to establish a systematic and rational framework for approaching shock that will inform your management.

Good critical care involves identifying a deficiency, applying an intervention, assessing the effect, and adjusting course. This is more relevant when it comes to shock than almost anything else. It is one thing to try to increase blood pressure in a patient with low blood pressure. It is quite another to identify that a patient is in shock with evidence of decreased oxygen delivery, to classify and diagnose the etiology of that shock, assessing the need for an intervention such as fluids or pressors aimed at correcting a deficiency, and witnessing the effect of that intervention.

By establishing this framework, we have an opportunity to determine what is missing in the resuscitation and ultimately consider how our interventions at the bedside are affecting care.

SUGGESTED READING

Hochman, J. S. (2003). Cardiogenic shock complicating acute myocardial infarction: expanding the paradigm. *Circulation*, *107*(24), 2998–3002.

Landry, D. W., & Oliver, J. A. (2001). The pathogenesis of vasodilatory shock. *The New England Journal of Medicine*, *345*(8), 588–595.

Monnet, X., Jabot, J., Maizel, J., Richard, C., & Teboul, J. L. (2011). Norepinephrine increases cardiac preload and reduces preload dependency assessed by passive leg raising in septic shock patients. *Critical Care Medicine*, *39*(4), 689–694.

Monnet, X., Letierce, A., Hamzaoui, O., Chemla, D., Anguel, N., Osman, D., et al. (2011). Arterial pressure allows monitoring the changes in cardiac output induced by volume expansion but not by norepinephrine. *Critical Care Medicine*, *39*(6), 1394–1399.

Richard, J. C., Bayle, F., Bourdin, G., Leray, V., Debord, S., Delannoy, B., et al. (2015). Preload dependence indices to titrate volume expansion during septic shock: a randomized controlled trial. *Critical Care*, *19*(1), 1–13.

Ventetuolo, C. E., & Klinger, J. R. (2014). Management of acute right ventricular failure in the intensive care unit. *Annals of the American Thoracic Society*, *11*(5), 811–822.

3

Recognition of Shock

Now we are going to bring our discussion of shock to the next level and start to explore some patterns that can help us with recognition of shock. Remember, if we no longer define shock as low blood pressure, we need to have some indicators to help us recognize what can be a startlingly subtle yet dangerous state.

But first, a caveat. Imagine you go to the beach one warm summer day. Even though it is a popular beach, you note that there are almost no people there. You notice a purple flag flying over the lifeguard stand. You then notice people running out of the water. Maybe this pattern means that there is something dangerous in the water. Or maybe it is just early in the day, most people haven't arrived yet, and the people running out of the water were just playing.

The point being that patterns can be helpful, but they can also be limiting. They don't always hold true, but they can give a framework for what to expect, especially if you have an appreciation for the limitations and exceptions.

That said, let's consider a pattern commonly seen in shock.

WHAT DOES SHOCK LOOK LIKE AT THE BEDSIDE?

Imagine you are receiving a patient in the intensive care unit (ICU). The team that is handing him off says, "I'm not sure what is going on with him, but he has us worried. We are thinking he may be in shock."

What might you expect this patient to look like over the next 12–24 hours assuming he continues to worsen? Not every presentation is the same, but the following is a pattern that is useful to consider (Fig. 3.1).

Let's consider each of these phases.

Phase 1: cardiac output compensation

Remember that as DO_2:VO_2 falls, the most ready way that the body can increase this is by augmenting cardiac output. Cardiac output increases when the stroke volume increases (heart squeezes harder) or heart rate increases (heart beats faster). In most people, this can augment CO, and consequently DO_2 several fold (up to 35-fold in some athletes).

Clinically, this can be manifested by tachycardia or by increased pulse pressure (the difference of systole and diastole) (Fig. 3.2).

Ultimately, if DO_2 is not able to keep up with VO_2 requirements, then the DO_2:VO_2 ratio starts to fall, manifested by lower venous oxygen saturation (Fig. 3.3).

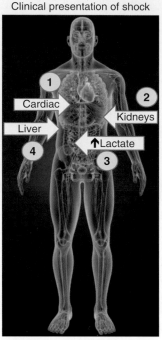

Clinical presentation of shock

Phase 1: Cardiac output
compensation

Phase 2: Decreased
renal function

Phase 2: Decreased
renal function

Phase 3: Lactic acidosis

Phase 4: Liver injury

FIG. 3.1 A commonly observed pattern in shock: augmentation of cardiac output, diminished renal function, lactic acidosis, and liver injury. (Modified from Sciencepics/Shutterstock.com.)

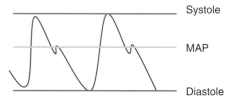

FIG. 3.2 Pulse pressure: the difference between systole and diastole. *MAP*, Mean arterial pressure.

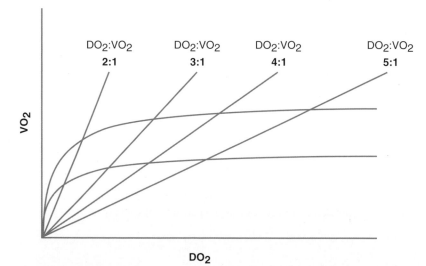

FIG. 3.3 Venous oxygen saturation and DO_2:VO_2.

When does this pattern not apply?

There are many reasons other than shock for the heart rate/cardiac output to be augmented in patients in the ICU (agitation, delirium, medication effect, withdrawal, etc.). However, a rise in these parameters should give pause and lead to the consideration that it may be compensation for a drop in DO_2.

Additionally, a venous oxygen saturation cannot always be used as a surrogate for $DO_2{:}VO_2$. We remember that if the VO_2 remains constant, a dropping venous oxygen saturation can be a surrogate for a drop in $DO_2{:}VO_2$.

However, what happens when the cardiac output remains in a high output state, say due to a catecholamine surge or in early sepsis? In this case, the blood may be circulated around the periphery so fast that the oxygen is unable to be extracted. This may lead to a higher than expected venous oxygen saturation, which may not correspond with adequate $DO_2{:}VO_2$.

In another example, as shock progresses, target organs may begin shutting down, leading to a decreased VO_2. This will lead to an elevated $DO_2{:}VO_2$ ratio that does not actually mean that the body is adequately delivering oxygen to meet the tissue needs, but rather may have a more ominous meaning (Fig. 3.4).

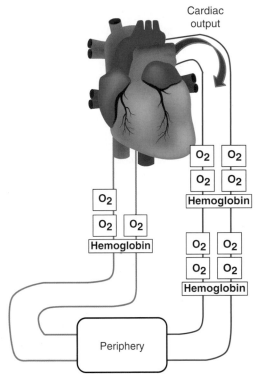

FIG. 3.4 High venous oxygen saturation as a consequence of decreased VO_2 in decompensated shock. (Modified from Ody_Stocker/Shutterstock.com.)

Phase 2: decreased renal function

As $DO_2{:}VO_2$ continues to fall, the renal function will often decline next, manifested by a drop in urine output and an eventual rise in creatinine (Fig. 3.5). This is due to a variety of mechanisms, some adaptive, some pathologic.

The adaptive component of this mechanism is a drop in urine output in response to a decrease in renal perfusion pressure. This has the additional effect of maintaining intravascular volume and augmenting preload. However, there can also be a pathologic mechanism, in which decreased

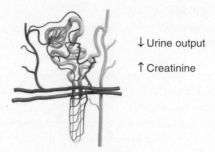

↓ Urine output

↑ Creatinine

FIG. 3.5 Renal effects of decreased perfusion. (Modified from Axel_Kock/Shutterstock.com.)

perfusion and shock state can cause damage to the renal glomerular architecture. This can be manifested as a worsening urine output and rising creatinine that does not improve after perfusion is restored.

Phase 3: lactic acidosis

Lactate level is a common test ordered to quantify patients in shock. The reason is that lactate is a marker of a transition from aerobic metabolism to anaerobic metabolism. Therefore, as $DO_2:VO_2$ continues to drop, the proportion of cells requiring anaerobic metabolism increases and lactic acid rises. This rise can be delayed and typically happens after the compensation in cardiac output and the decline of renal function.

Does an elevated lactate always mean a patient is in shock?

To better understand how to interpret a lactic acid level in shock, let's go all the way down to the cellular level and consider how glucose is metabolized.

Glucose is transported into the cell via the GLUT4 receptor and enters the cytoplasm. It is then phosphorylated and catalyzed by the enzyme G6PD. The phosphorylated glucose is then split into pyruvate generating adenosine triphosphate (ATP). Pyruvate is then transported into the mitochondria via the enzyme pyruvate dehydrogenase.

Once in the mitochondria, the pyruvate is used to generate ATP via the electron transport chain with oxygen playing a central role by being the final electron acceptor (Fig. 3.6).

Stay with me! There is a reason for every receptor and enzyme that was just mentioned.

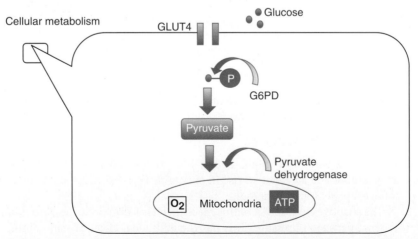

FIG. 3.6 Normal metabolism of glucose. *ATP,* Adenosine triphosphate.

What happens if there is no oxygen? (Decreased $DO_2{:}VO_2$)

If there is a decreased $DO_2{:}VO_2$, then pyruvate accumulates and it is metabolized into lactate (Fig. 3.7). This forms the basis for the assumption that lactic acidosis is an indicator of shock. Since it takes time for reserves to be depleted and for cells to shift to this anaerobic metabolism, this lactic acidosis usually occurs on the order of hours, rather than the seconds as seen for cardiac compensation and the minutes seen for renal compensation.

Ok, so the higher the lactate, the worse the $DO_2{:}VO_2$, right?

This is the theory to some degree, but again, we need to understand when it works and when it breaks down. Let's explore further.

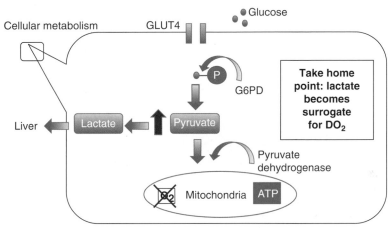

FIG. 3.7 Impaired oxygen delivery and the production of lactate. *ATP,* Adenosine triphosphate.

When elevated lactate does not necessarily mean a deficiency in $DO_2{:}VO_2$

Let's examine when lactate level may not necessarily correspond to a deficiency in DO_2 (or at the very least, when augmenting DO_2 may not necessarily lead to a **clearance** of lactate). As an example, let's consider septic shock.

In sepsis, there may be a variety of derangements to include hypoglycemia, downregulation of GLUT4 through catecholamine administration, decreased availability of phosphorous, and decreased activity of pyruvate dehydrogenase. All of these derangements may contribute to altered levels of pyruvate in the cytoplasm of cells of septic patients, independent of oxygen delivery/availability. Coupled with liver injury, which can also predominate in sepsis, you can imagine how elevated lactate/impaired lactate clearance can occur, even in the setting of adequate oxygen delivery (Fig. 3.8).

Phase 4: liver injury

Liver injury is the fourth phase of shock that can be very revealing. While augmentation of cardiac output (phase 1) can occur in a matter of seconds, decreased renal function can occur in a matter of minutes, and lactic acidosis can occur over the course of hours, liver injury usually becomes apparent over the next 1–2 days.

The pattern is usually a precipitous rise in aspartate aminotransferase/alanine aminotransferase (AST/ALT) over the course of a few days. In severe shock, these values may elevate to the thousands in the first day or so, with improvement after the shock is addressed. In the same way that elevation of liver function tests can be delayed in shock liver, the improvement in these parameters can also be delayed after the cause of shock is resolved.

The process can be subtle and difficult to pick up. For example, there are other causes of elevated liver function tests in patients with shock, such as sepsis itself, right heart dysfunction with

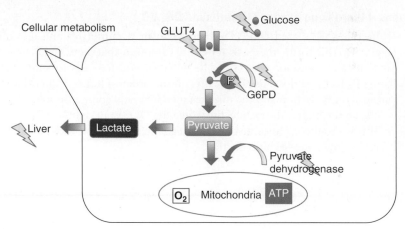

FIG. 3.8 Impaired glucose metabolism and increased lactate production in sepsis. *ATP*, Adenosine triphosphate.

congestion of blood in liver, acalculous cholecystitis, and medication effects. Shock liver can often be distinguished from these other causes of liver injury by the degree of elevation of liver function tests, but this is not always the case. Liver injury in the setting of shock should always be put in the appropriate clinical context.

PUTTING IT ALL TOGETHER

Shock can be overt in its presentation or very subtle. Regardless, time is often of the essence – even small delays in the recognition of shock can lead to a downward spiral that can be difficult to reverse. In the next chapter, we explore the importance of assessing the cause of decompensation and quantifying the response of the patient to our interventions. Early and accurate recognition will be an essential part of this process.

SUGGESTED READING

Birgens, H. S., Henriksen, J., Matzen, P., & Poulsen, H. (1978). The shock liver: clinical and biochemical findings in patients with centrilobular liver necrosis following cardiogenic shock. *Acta Medica Scandinavica*, *204*(1–6), 417–421.

Cecconi, M., De Backer, D., Antonelli, M., Beale, R., Bakker, J., & Hofer, C., et al. (2014). Consensus on circulatory shock and hemodynamic monitoring. Task force of the European Society of Intensive Care Medicine. *Intensive Care Medicine*, *40*(12), 1795–1815.

Garcia-Alvarez, M., Marik, P., & Bellomo, R. (2014). Sepsis-associated hyperlactatemia. *Critical care*, *18*(5), 1–11.

Marik, P. E., & Bellomo, R. (2013). Lactate clearance as a target of therapy in sepsis: a flawed paradigm. *OA Critical Care*, *1*(1), 3.

Marik, P. E., Cavallazzi, R., Vasu, T., & Hirani, A. (2009). Dynamic changes in arterial waveform derived variables and fluid responsiveness in mechanically ventilated patients: a systematic review of the literature. *Critical Care Medicine*, *37*(9), 2642–2647.

Rhodes, A., Boussat, S., Chemla, D., Anguel, N., Mercat, A., & Lecarpentier, Y., et al. (2000). Relation between respiratory changes in arterial pulse pressure and fluid responsiveness in septic patients with acute circulatory failure. *American Journal of Respiratory and Critical Care Medicine*, *162*(1), 134–138.

Rhodes, A., Evans, L. E., Alhazzani, W., Levy, M. M., Antonelli, M., & Ferrer, R., et al. (2017). Surviving sepsis campaign: international guidelines for management of sepsis and septic shock: 2016. *Intensive Care Medicine*, *43*(3), 304–377.

4

Hypoxia

Hopefully by now we are starting to develop a healthy appreciation for oxygen delivery – why it is so important, how it can be augmented, and the limitations that exist. We have also discussed that when this process starts to break down (i.e., when oxygen delivery is compromised in cardiac/respiratory failure), we must optimize oxygen delivery through critical care interventions, which can come with a cost.

Let's briefly return to our consideration of oxygen delivery and hemoglobin binding. In Chapter 1, we explored how oxygen would bind to hemoglobin and how important the oxygenated hemoglobin molecule was to the delivery of oxygen. Now we will explore what happens when there is less oxygen readily available to be able to bind and saturate hemoglobin (Fig. 4.1).

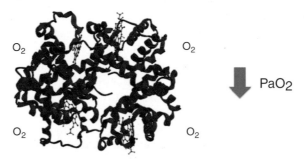

FIG. 4.1 Saturation of hemoglobin requires adequate PaO_2. (Modified from Raimundo79/Shutterstock.com.)

HOW DOES OXYGEN ENTER THE BODY?

Take a deep breath in. Go ahead, I'll wait … now let it out. What is happening when we do this simple function? With every breath in and every breath out, we are allowing oxygen to enter our body, we are enabling the delivery and use of that oxygen, and we are expiring carbon dioxide, the byproduct of that metabolism. This happens like clockwork, hundreds of times per hour, every day, whether we are conscious of it or not. None of this would be possible if there was not a ready and efficient way for oxygen to enter the body and carbon dioxide to exit.

To explore how this happens, follow that breath of air in – through the airway, past the bronchi, through the bronchioles, all the way down until we get to the level of the alveoli. It is at this level that gas exchange between the lungs and the blood is able to happen in an efficient manner, by setting up an interface between the blood vessels and the alveoli.

Due to the close proximity of the blood and the alveoli, this interface allows for diffusion of gases down their respective concentration gradients. Just like if you dropped a drop of dye into a glass of water, diffusion allows molecules to go from areas of high concentration to areas of low concentration. It is this diffusion gradient that drives the flow of oxygen and carbon dioxide in such a manner that oxygen is able to enter the body and carbon dioxide is able to leave the body (Fig. 4.2).

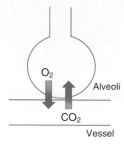

FIG. 4.2 O_2 and CO_2 diffusion at the blood-alveolar interface.

It is important to separate these two components of respiration out (ventilation of the alveoli and perfusion of the blood vessels) because they become vital to our discussion and allow us to better identify the level of the deficiency.

WHEN THE SYSTEM BREAKS DOWN

There are a host of reasons for low concentrations of oxygen in the blood. These can include hypoventilation, low inspired FiO_2, as is seen at high altitude, and diffusion defects where there is a breakdown at the level of the interstitium. The purpose of our discussion is to better understand the two components of the alveolar-blood interface, and how they interact with each other.

Deficiency at the level of the alveolus is labeled V by convention, whereas deficiency at the level of blood to perfuse the alveolus is labeled Q. If both are equally contributing to gas exchange, then the ratio of V/Q is equal to 1 (Fig. 4.3).

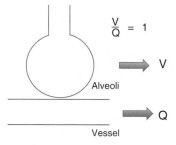

FIG. 4.3 Ventilation perfusion matching.

When there is a deficiency of one relative to the other, there is V/Q mismatch. Let's look at two permutations.

In Chapter 2, we described in detail the specifics of when and how the right heart can fail. Now let's consider the effect of a decline in right heart function on respiratory function.

If there is a decline in the right ventricular function, the overall perfusion to the alveolar-blood vessel apparatus will decline. That means that on some level, whether just through decreased perfusion or the total lack of perfusion, there will be V/Q > 1. This manifests as an alveolar unit where is fully ventilated but does not participate in gas exchange. It is as if there is no connection between the two – air comes in and out with no improvement in ventilation. This is referred to as "dead space" (Fig. 4.4).

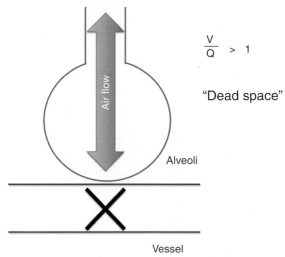

$$\frac{V}{Q} > 1$$

"Dead space"

FIG. 4.4 Schematic for dead space

Let's contrast this with the opposite scenario, where V/Q < 1. This would correspond with any time when there is decreased ability of air to enter into the alveolar component of the alveolar-blood vessel interface – pneumonia, edema, mucous plugging, etc. In this case, blood traverses across the interface with no ability for gas to diffuse. In this manner, this is referred to as "shunt" (Fig. 4.5).

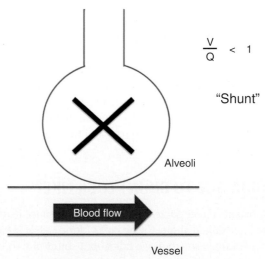

$$\frac{V}{Q} < 1$$

"Shunt"

FIG. 4.5 Schematic for shunt

Although the temptation is to think of the lungs as a homogenous collection of alveoli and the pulmonary circulation similarly as a uniform collection of blood vessels perfusing these alveoli, the situation can be quite complex. There can be areas of the lung with profound V/Q mismatch, such as complete collapse of one lobe of the lung due to mucous plug, for example. In this case, the collapsed area of the lung may have a V/Q much less than 1, while the remainder of the lung may have normal matching of ventilation to perfusion.

Consider also that even under normal conditions, blood tends to be gravity dependent leading to increased distension of the pulmonary blood vessels in the lower portions of the lung (and thus V/Q < 1), while alveoli may be more distended in the upper areas of the lungs (with V/Q > 1) (Fig. 4.6).

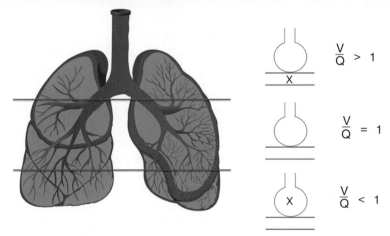

FIG 4.6 Variation in ventilation and perfusion matching in normal lungs. (Modified from YanGe_Tam/Shutterstock.com.)

So why make this distinction?

We distinguish aberrations in the V/Q matching in this way, because the physiology is very different. Just like the models for shock, this classification should help to develop an approach for thinking about respiratory failure, which can then be built upon. Specifically, let's examine the case of hypoxia and the role of mechanical ventilation.

There are many reasons to undergo mechanical ventilation – inability to protect airway, excessive secretions, expected clinical course, etc. However, in order to best understand the breakdown of the delivery of oxygen due to respiratory failure, we will focus our discussion on the role of mechanical ventilation on improving hypoxia due to shunt, where V/Q is less than 1. Let's now focus in on shunt, its specific physiology, and the role of mechanical ventilation in mitigating the ensuing hypoxia.

WHAT DOES HYPOXIA DUE TO SHUNT LOOK LIKE?

Shunt is important to recognize and understand because its physiology is unique.

While we have talked about the alveolar-blood vessel interface as one unit, there are millions of alveoli in the lungs, so when we talk about shunt physiology, we are acknowledging that this physiology exists as a spectrum, becoming more profound as more shunting occurs.

Let's start by understanding what happens with normal lungs, with minimal shunt. If no shunt exists, every alveoli is paired with a perfusing blood vessel and the maximum interface between those two is maintained. If you were to spread out the surface area of this interface, it would be the size of a tennis court, so you can quickly understand how the lungs can be so efficient at allowing oxygen to diffuse into the blood.

Not only are our hypothetical lungs with no shunt able to allow for a higher diffusion of oxygen at room air, but when we add higher concentration of inspired oxygen (FiO_2), we really start to see the difference. Because there is so much more area for oxygen to diffuse across, increasing the FiO_2 by a multiple of two-, three-, or fourfold not only increases the amount of oxygen that diffuses across but it does so at an exponential rate.

Now, let's consider what happens when there is 10% shunt. In this case, there is a slightly lower amount of oxygen that can diffuse across at room air, as noted by the lower PaO_2. However, as we increase the FiO_2, say from 2 L nasal cannula to 6 L to a non-rebreather face mask, there is going to be an increase in PaO_2 of the blood almost as high if there was no shunt – however, notice that it takes a higher FiO_2 to get there!

As the amount of shunt progresses, notice that it not only corresponds to a lower initial PaO_2 at room air but also to a more shallow slope of the line, with decreasing gains in PaO_2 for every escalation in FiO_2 (Fig. 4.7).

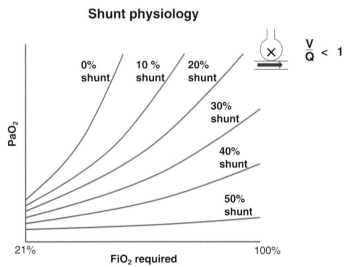

FIG 4.7 Shunt physiology and the relation of PaO_2 to FiO_2

Notice what happens when we arrive at approximately 50% shunt. At this point, you can observe that the curve is essentially flat. This means that no matter how much oxygen you give, there will be no subsequent increase in oxygen that diffuses along to the blood. This pattern is what is meant when we say "shunt physiology" – the point where adding more inspired oxygen will not help increase the blood oxygen concentration, no matter how much is given (Fig. 4.8).

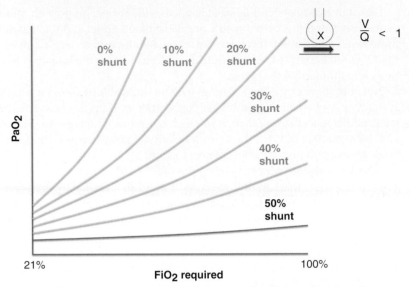

FIG. 4.8 Unresponsiveness to FiO_2 increases with progression of shunt

Why is this?

Imagine you are driving down a road where the speed limit is 30 miles per hour. You don't want to get caught speeding, so you set your speed at 30 miles per hour. You then pass a sign that says the speed limit is now 40 miles per hour. You can now increase your speed to 40 miles per hour.

However, now imagine that you are traveling behind a truck that is going 30 miles an hour. You pass the sign that the speed limit is 40 miles an hour; however, the truck continues driving at 30 miles an hour. Assuming you cannot pass the truck, your speed has to stay at 30 miles per hour.

The same is true of FiO_2 with shunt. The higher the FiO_2 the more oxygen comes across the alveolar-blood interface. However, when alveoli are shunted, the actual inspired amount of oxygen is inconsequential, just like the speed limit is inconsequential if you are stuck behind another car (Fig. 4.7).

So that's it? Game over?

Not necessarily. It just means that we have to improve the shunt fraction if we want to improve the overall oxygenation.

Let's imagine that you are caring for a patient with pneumonia who has become progressively hypoxic over the last several hours. You have witnessed the PaO_2 (and oxygen saturation) continue to decline despite increasing FiO_2 levels, as you have progressed from nasal cannula to non-rebreather. What do you do next?

As you have intuitively come up with, the next step is consideration for intubation. Let's look at why intubation (and positive pressure) improves oxygenation.

IMPACT OF POSITIVE PRESSURE ON HYPOXIA DUE TO SHUNT

Although we initially started discussing shunt as a mismatch between the alveolar unit (V) and the vascular unit (Q), in reality, the lungs exist as a heterogeneous collection of alveoli, which exist in various phases of collapse and inflation.

Positive pressure further inflates the lungs. It pushes air into the lungs, allowing for alveoli that are not open to inflate. This allows for recruitment of alveoli that are not participating in gas exchange (Fig. 4.9A,B).

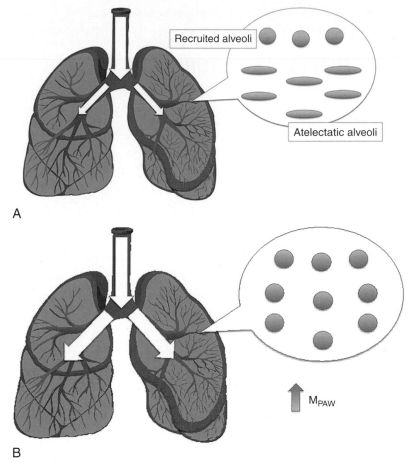

FIG. 4.9 (A) and (B) Positive pressure and alveolar recruitment. M_{PAW}, Mean airway pressure. (Modified from YanGe_Tam/Shutterstock.com.)

WHAT IS THE MEAN AIRWAY PRESSURE AND HOW CAN WE AUGMENT IT?

When a breath is delivered from a ventilator, there is a specific amount of pressure that is exhibited at the beginning of a breath and a higher amount of pressure that is exhibited at the end of the breath. The mean pressure is the average pressure exerted between these two pressures and ultimately affects what is exerted on the alveoli. The higher the mean airway pressure, the higher the pressure that can be exerted to open recruitable alveoli (to a point).

The mean airway pressure is ultimately determined by the pressure at the beginning and end of the breath as well as the time spent during inspiration and exhalation, according to the following relationship:

$$M_{PAW} = \frac{(T_I \times P_{IP}) + (T_E \times PEEP)}{T_I + T_E}$$

Where M_{PAW} is the mean airway pressure, P_{IP} is the inspiratory pressure, PEEP is the positive end expiratory pressure, T_I is the time of inspiration, and T_E is the time of expiration.

Since the time of exhalation is greater than the time of inhalation, augmentation of PEEP is the most ready way to augment the mean airway pressure and, by extension, improve shunt and oxygenation.

WHAT ARE THE EFFECTS OF INCREASING PEEP?

Let's envision that shunt continues to worsen on mechanical ventilation, leading us to increase PEEP in order to augment mean airway pressure and recruit additional alveoli into gas exchange. What is the effect of this?

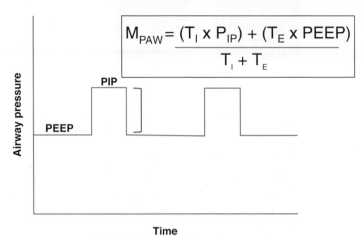

$$M_{PAW} = \frac{(T_I \times P_{IP}) + (T_E \times PEEP)}{T_I + T_E}$$

FIG. 4.10 Airway pressure over time

Let's look at the graph in Fig. 4.10, comparing airway pressure over time for a patient on positive pressure ventilation.

You will notice that all airway pressures are positive, with airway pressure going from a low point during the end of expiration (PEEP) to a high point during inspiration (PIP). The difference between these two pressures is the amount of pressure that is delivered with each breath, or the driving pressure.

Now let's explore increasing PEEP. Increasing PEEP will raise the baseline and increase the overall mean airway pressure. However, the effect of doing so may be that either the difference between the two pressures decreases or that the inspiratory pressure must increase if you want to maintain the same driving pressure.

WHAT ARE THE EFFECTS OF WORSENING COMPLIANCE?

This effect on the overall inspiratory pressures becomes more pronounced as compliance worsens. What causes compliance to worsen? Take your pick – inflammation/acute respiratory distress syndrome (ARDS), edema, mucous plugging, atelectasis, pneumonia, etc. Either way, as the alveolar unit becomes progressively flooded and collapsed, two adverse effects occur: the shunt worsens and the lungs become less likely to expand with any breath. Imagine trying to blow up a balloon right out of the package versus one that has been stretched out. The relationship between pressure delivered and compliance is as follows:

$$Compliance = \frac{\Delta Volume}{\Delta Pressure}$$

Which in the context of mechanical ventilation can be rewritten as:

$$Compliance = \frac{V_T}{PIP - PEEP}$$

Where V_T is the tidal volume, or the total volume delivered with each breath.

As compliance decreases, this means that only two things can happen with regards to this relationship – either higher driving pressures have to be used to maintain the same tidal volume, or you will observe lower tidal volume at the same driving pressure.

Maintaining an adequate tidal volume becomes essential, as it is one of the two variables determining the clearance of CO_2, with the following relationship:

$$Minute\ Ventilation = V_T \times Respiratory\ Rate$$

THE CHALLENGING TRADEOFF OF WORSENING RESPIRATORY FAILURE

Now you are faced with a difficult tradeoff that often comes up as lungs become progressively compromised. You have to maintain adequate mean airway pressures to allow for oxygenation, but this may lead to either higher inspiratory airway pressures or decreased tidal volume. Higher inspiratory airway pressures will eventually damage the lungs (called barotrauma) and worsen mortality, while lower tidal volumes will lead to a lower minute ventilation and worsening CO_2 clearance. This can be initially mitigated by increasing the respiratory rate to a point but, eventually, you are faced with the situation where you are faced with worsening oxygenation/ventilation or potentially damaging the lungs with higher settings.

PUTTING IT TOGETHER

Maintaining adequate levels of diffused oxygen in the blood is essential for hemoglobin to adequately saturate. Without well-saturated hemoglobin, oxygen delivery becomes a progressively tenuous proposition.

While there are many causes of hypoxia, shunt is an important cause, as there is a limited effect of increasing inspired oxygen (FiO_2). Rather, alveolar units must be recruited through increasing the mean airway pressure. However, as respiratory failure continues to worsen, with progression of shunt fraction and worsening compliance, the choice sometimes becomes either accepting worsening parameters of oxygenation/ventilation or subjecting the lungs to more damaging effects as we continue to increase the "dose" of mechanical ventilation. We will further explore the effects of how we "dose" mechanical ventilation and other critical care interventions in the next chapter.

SUGGESTED READING

Benatar, S. R., Hewlett, A. M., & Nunn, J. F. (1973). The use of iso-shunt lines for control of oxygen therapy. *British Journal of Anaesthesia*, 45(7), 711–718.

Doorduin, J., Nollet, J. L., Vugts, M. P., Roesthuis, L. H., Akankan, F., & van der Hoeven, J. G., et al. (2016). Assessment of dead-space ventilation in patients with acute respiratory distress syndrome: a prospective observational study. *Critical Care*, 20(1), 1–10.

Henderson, W. R., & Sheel, A. W. (2012). Pulmonary mechanics during mechanical ventilation. *Respiratory Physiology & Neurobiology*, 180(2-3), 162–172.

Hess, D. R. (2015). Recruitment maneuvers and PEEP titration. *Respiratory Care, 60*(11), 1688–1704.

Malhotra, A. (2007). Low-tidal-volume ventilation in the acute respiratory distress syndrome. *New England Journal of Medicine, 357*(11), 1113–1120.

Marini, J. J., & Ravenscraft, S. A. (1992). Mean airway pressure: physiologic determinants and clinical importance—Part 1: physiologic determinants and measurements. *Critical Care Medicine, 20*(10), 1461–1472.

Mercat, A., Richard, J. C., Vielle, B., Jaber, S., Osman, D., Diehl, J. L., et al. (2008). Positive end-expiratory pressure setting in adults with acute lung injury and acute respiratory distress syndrome: a randomized controlled trial. *JAMA, 299*(6), 646–655.

West, J. B. (2012). *Respiratory physiology: The Essentials*. Lippincott Williams & Wilkins.

5

The Failure of DO$_2$ – Did What I Do to the Patient Just Work?

By now, I wouldn't be surprised if you were asking yourself, "I thought this was a book about ECMO?" Why are we talking about hemoglobin dissociation, shock recognition, shunt physiology, and lactate clearance?

Hopefully this chapter will put it all together.

We have been building toward a fundamental concept that we will unpack more in this chapter, namely, that everything we do in the intensive care unit (ICU) comes with a cost. There is toxicity associated with interventions, and this toxicity is often dose related.

Let me underscore that one more time, to hopefully make sure we appreciate its implications.

Every intervention in the ICU has a dose-related toxicity – the more we have to dial up support, the more we have to consider the potentially toxic effects of what we are doing (Fig. 5.1).

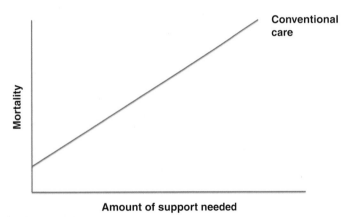

FIG. 5.1 The dose-related toxicity of conventional care

Let's return to the oxygen delivery equation:

$$DO_2 \rightarrow CO \times Hb \times SaO_2$$

We are going to unpack the concept of dose-related toxicity for each component, highlighting the cost of optimizing each component, especially as things start to break down as patients begin to decompensate.

WHAT IS MEANT BY DOSE-RELATED TOXICITY OF ICU INTERVENTIONS?

Let's say you have a patient who is septic from a urinary tract infection, with *Escherichia coli*, a gram-negative bacteria, growing in the urine as well as blood cultures. He is placed on vancomycin, an antibiotic with gram-positive coverage but poor gram-negative coverage. When he does not improve, the dose of vancomycin is increased 20-fold.

What is wrong with this story? Why do we all cringe at this plan?

There are two fundamental flaws to this plan:

1. You have to know what you are treating
2. If you are treating the wrong diagnosis, increasing the dose will only expose this patient to toxicity without any benefit

IS THIS REALLY A FAIR EXAMPLE?

Let's entertain another example. In this case, it is a patient who arrives in the ICU with shock due to a pulmonary embolism with primarily right ventricular failure. The team assesses the patient, sees a low blood pressure, high heart rate, and low urine output and gives fluid.

When this doesn't work, they give another bolus of fluid. And then a third.

After this doesn't work, they initiate norepinephrine, with no improvement in blood pressure, uptitrating from 0.1 mcg/kg/min to the maximum of 2 mcg/kg/min. After this doesn't work, the team initiates vasopressin, uptitrated to a maximum rate of 0.04 units/min. After this, with the patient still hypotensive, the team initiates a neosynephrine drip, uptitrating it to a maximum of 200 mcg/kg/min.

WHAT IS HAPPENING WITH THIS PATIENT?

Much like our first patient who was being treated with escalating doses of the wrong antibiotic, this patient was exposed to escalating doses of support that was not helping his underlying condition. Let's explore why.

In a pulmonary embolism, there is an occlusive thrombus in the pulmonary artery, which can increase right ventricular afterload and lead to right heart failure.

Recall from Chapter 2 that preload has a limited effect on a failing right ventricle. This is due to the various characteristics of the right ventricle – it is less muscular, shortens on a different axis, and this is eventually limited by the pericardium (Fig. 5.2).

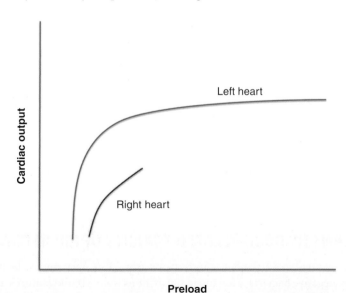

FIG. 5.2 Preload responsiveness for the left and right heart

Additionally, recall that the failing right ventricle will not only dilate but can actually compress on the left ventricle, as is illustrated here. This can be the unfortunate consequence of excessive fluid bolus in right heart failure (Fig. 5.3).

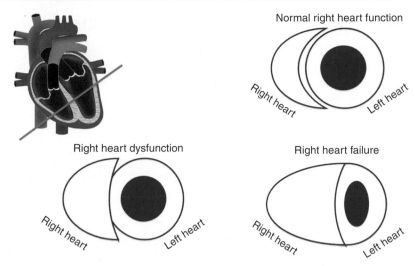

FIG. 5.3 The effect of excessive preload on a failing right ventricle. (Modified from Ody_Stocker/Shutterstock.com.)

Next, the team initiates norepinephrine, which has the effect of improving systemic vascular resistance by increasing vasoconstriction, but remember also increases the pulmonary vascular resistance, which will only worsen right ventricular afterload (Fig. 5.4).

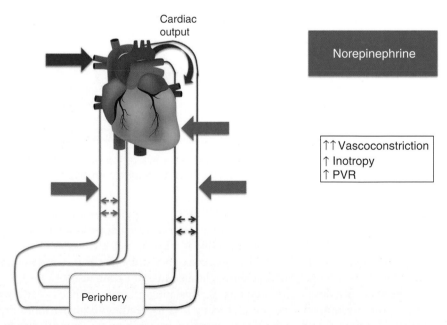

FIG. 5.4 Effect of norepinephrine on pulmonary vascular resistance. *PVR*, Pulmonary vascular resistance. (Modified from Ody_Stocker/Shutterstock.com.)

Uptitrating norepinephrine and neosynephrine was the equivalent of increasing vancomycin to 20 g – uptitrating a medication that is not improving the clinical situation while only causing more adverse effects.

HOW DO PRESSORS WORSEN THE CLINICAL SITUATION IN SHOCK?

One of the most important clinical effects of a mean arterial pressure (MAP) is maintaining a vascular pressure head to allow forward flow of blood and perfusion of peripheral tissues and end organs.

This pressure differential is normally maintained by the higher pressure that exists in the arterial system versus the venous system, which drives blood forward. The lower the MAP, the lower this forward flow and the lower the perfusion of the end organs (Fig. 5.5).

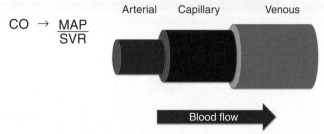

FIG. 5.5 The role of vascular tone in maintaining the vascular pressure head. *CO*, Cardiac output; *MAP*, mean arterial pressure; *SVR*, systemic vascular resistance

Think of a garden hose that is losing water flow, not allowing you to reach a bush that you are watering. You can put your thumb over the top, which increases the pressure differential and allows you to now reach that bush. However, if the water flow continues to decrease, further occluding the hose with your thumb may allow you to reach the bush, but the overall amount of water that is reaching the bush decreases (Fig. 5.6).

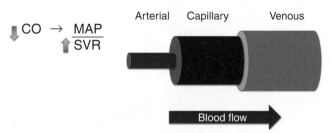

FIG. 5.6 The effect of maintaining mean arterial pressure through vasopressors on forward blood flow. *CO*, Cardiac output; *MAP*, mean arterial pressure; *SVR*, systemic vascular resistance

The same phenomenon occurs when pressors are applied in the setting of decreasing cardiac output. They can be used to a point to maintain this vascular pressure differential, but eventually, the effect is that the overall delivery of blood/oxygen is decreased. This is why you can maintain an adequate MAP with escalating pressors but still experience worsening markers of shock (decreased urine output, lactic acidosis, elevated liver function tests).

The effect is a dose-related response of escalating pressors in shock – with worsening clinical effects, diminishing returns, and increasing toxicity, leading to higher mortality with escalating pressor requirements/dosages. By the time you are reaching for your third or fourth pressor, the expected mortality of your patient has risen precipitously (Fig. 5.7).

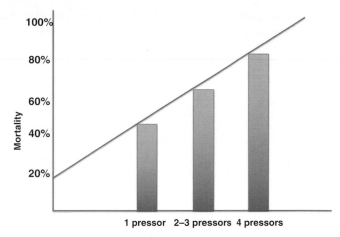

FIG. 5.7 Mortality associated with vasopressor use in cardiogenic shock

This is not to just say that patients who require more pressors are also those more likely to die. It is also saying that when pressors reach escalating dosages, there is less of a chance of them achieving adequate perfusion, and may actually make things worse, leading to the downward spiral of shock.

HOW DO I PREVENT THE DOWNWARD SPIRAL OF SHOCK?

This downward spiraling with interventions making things worse rather than better is a disturbing proposition. Like most downward spirals, the cause comes from not knowing where the spiral is heading and how to counteract. Therefore, let's propose the following stepwise approach, which is designed for assessment of the clinical situation, observation of the effects, and realignment if necessary:

1. Have a diagnosis of shock (obstructive, cardiogenic, distributive, hypovolemic).
2. Implicate a cause of this type of shock (vasodilatory shock due to sepsis due to pneumonia v. obstructive shock due to PE as examples).
3. Address the shock diagnosis with a targeted intervention.
4. Observe the effect of that intervention. Did it improve some parameter or worsen it?

If by step 4 you are not feeling more reassured, then start over and reassess what is going on with the patient.

How Does This Downward Spiral Apply to the Other Components of the Oxygen Delivery Equation?

Returning again to our oxygen delivery equation:

$$DO_2 \rightarrow CO \times Hb \times SaO_2$$

In a similar way that we talked about how attempts to optimize cardiac output can lead to toxicity, let's now review how optimizing SaO_2 can lead to toxicity.

Like we discussed in Chapter 4, oxygen is able to enter the body efficiently through the alveolar-blood interface and the ability of O_2 to diffuse down its concentration gradient. However, as the degree of shunt progresses (whether due to worsening pulmonary edema, pneumonia, atelectasis, mucous plugging, etc.), this diffusion gradient becomes not only progressively difficult to maintain but also cannot be improved by the amount of oxygen administered, as illustrated in Fig. 5.8.

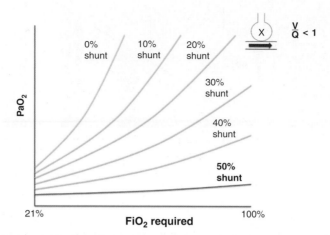

FIG. 5.8 Progressive shunt leading to lower oxygen diffusion despite escalating oxygen administration

At this point, the way to improve oxygenation is to allow for better recruitment of alveoli through augmentation of mean airway pressure.

So to review, the two ways to improve the amount of oxygen that diffuses into the blood from the lungs are to increase the amount of oxygen and to augment the mean airway pressure. Now let's unpack these two strategies, this time with extra attention on the adverse effect of doing so.

WHY IS INCREASING THE AMOUNT OF OXYGEN HARMFUL?

It seems like one of the simplest interventions we can do – if a patient has low oxygen saturations, we increase the amount of oxygen they are receiving. However, oxygen itself can be toxic, especially as concentrations increase. Besides the harmful effects of oxygen administration at the cellular level due to increased free radicals there is a harmful effect of increased oxygen concentrations at the blood-alveolar interface that is worth exploring.

As oxygen concentration increases, this increases the relative concentration of O_2 molecules in the alveolus relative to other gases, mainly nitrogen (N_2). Because oxygen exists at a higher concentration in the alveolus relative to the blood, it always diffuses down its concentration gradient (Fig. 5.9).

N_2 does not have this gradient and therefore does not diffuse. Thus, the higher the concentration of O_2, the more likely for all of the contents of the alveolus to diffuse into the blood and cause collapse of the alveolar unit (Fig. 5.10).

HARMFUL EFFECTS OF RAISING MEAN AIRWAY PRESSURE

Remember that as shunt increased, the way to improve overall oxygenation becomes dependent on the ability to recruit additional alveoli, by raising the mean airway pressure, mainly through increasing positive end-expiratory pressure (PEEP), as there is more time spent in expiration than in inspiration as illustrated in Fig. 5.11.

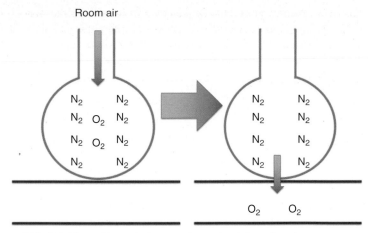

FIG. 5.9 The effect of nitrogen in maintaining alveolar patency

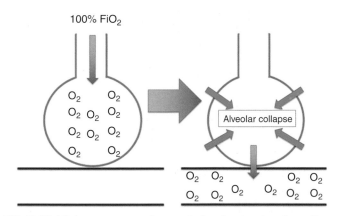

FIG. 5.10 High oxygen requirements leading to alveolar collapse

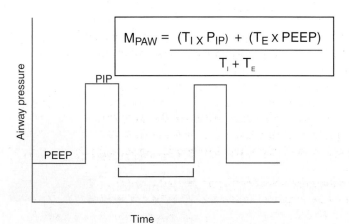

$$M_{PAW} = \frac{(T_I \times P_{IP}) + (T_E \times PEEP)}{T_I + T_E}$$

FIG. 5.11 The effect of PEEP on mean airway pressure due to longer time of expiration. *PEEP*, Peak end-expiratory pressure; *PIP*, peak inspiratory pressure

However, doing so has the adverse effect of increasing the overall pressure or decreasing the driving pressure. This is exacerbated as the overall pulmonary compliance decreases due to worsening progression of respiratory disease, whether due to edema, infection, inflammation/acute respiratory distress syndrome, plugging, etc. (Fig. 5.12).

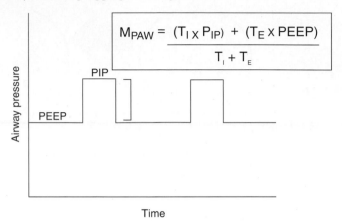

$$M_{PAW} = \frac{(T_I \times P_{IP}) + (T_E \times PEEP)}{T_I + T_E}$$

FIG. 5.12 The effect of raising PEEP on overall airway pressures. *PEEP*, Peak end-expiratory pressure; *PIP*, peak inspiratory pressure

As compliance starts to worsen, the overall driving pressure either has to increase or the tidal volume and PEEP has to decrease. The consequence is a worsening of oxygenation and ventilation/CO_2 removal (due to lower PEEP/tidal volume) or higher ventilator pressures have to be maintained, putting the patient at risk for worsening damage from the ventilator. The worsening of oxygenation/ventilation can exacerbate acidosis and vasodilation, increase right heart afterload, and lead to progressive myocardial depression, all with the downstream effect of decreasing cardiac output and further reduction of oxygen delivery.

WHAT ABOUT HEMOGLOBIN?

What about hemoglobin, our efficient compound that increases the delivery of oxygen so precipitously? Can we use hemoglobin to augment oxygen delivery?

$$DO_2 \rightarrow CO \times Hb \times SaO_2$$

It makes intuitive sense, especially if hemoglobin levels are low. If we are having difficulty delivering oxygen through a depressed cardiac output or inability to maintain saturations, why don't we just put more proverbial trucks on the road (Fig. 5.13)?

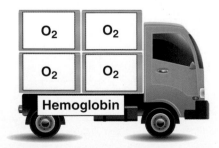

FIG. 5.13 Hemoglobin as a means for augmenting delivery of oxygen.
(From Bannosuke/Shutterstock.com.)

Unfortunately, like all the interventions that we have explored, hemoglobin augmentation through blood transfusion is subject to both diminishing returns with progressive administration, as well as toxicity that increases with progressive administration.

The diminishing returns center on the limitations of blood transfusion – the reality that transfused blood does not carry and deliver oxygen to the same degree that native blood does.

Additionally, there exist a multitude of toxicities that are well described with blood – including inflammatory effects, volume effects, and association with immune depressions and infections. These can impact organs throughout the body.

THE FINAL POINT...

Hopefully this chapter endows you with a sense of the dose-related response of critical care interventions designed to augment the delivery of oxygen. To be able to properly titrate the amount of support needed, we need to first understand the physiology of what is going on with the patient, what is deficient, and how we can support that deficiency in a way that is as effective and associated with as little toxicity as possible.

Realizing the toxicity of progressive uptitration of supportive care is an essential part of understanding the role of extracorporeal support. This is because, as we will now uncover, it is understanding the role of extracorporeal support in sparing this toxicity that will form the basis of how we approach extracorporeal membrane oxygenation (ECMO) and the role of ECMO in the care of critically ill patients.

Let's return now to our initial graph, showing the dose-related response of support with mortality, this time superimposing a proposed relationship that exists for specific patients who are now supported on ECMO, as represented by the green line (Fig. 5.14).

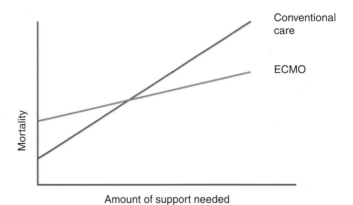

FIG. 5.14 ECMO as a potential option for decreasing the toxicity of high-dose critical care support

What if there is an intervention that we can do that can curb the toxicity of what we are doing to support our patients? What if that intervention involved more risk, cost, and expertise? Would it be worth it? As you can see, this intervention called ECMO, which we will spend the remainder of the book exploring and understanding, can only be useful if it is helping with the fundamental need of allowing for a sparing of toxicity, morbidity, and mortality, in order to offer the possibility of a better outcome for patients.

SUGGESTED READING

Beard, D. A., & Feigl, E. O. (2011). Understanding Guyton's venous return curves. *American Journal of Physiology-Heart and Circulatory Physiology, 301*(3), H629–H633.

Frank, L., Bucher, J. R., & Roberts, R. J. (1978). Oxygen toxicity in neonatal and adult animals of various species. *Journal of Applied Physiology: Respiratory, Environmental and Exercise Physiology, 45*, 699–704.

Griffith, D. E., Garcia, J. G., James, H. L., Callahan, K. S., Iriana, S., & Holiday, D. (1992). Hyperoxic exposure in humans: effects of 50 percent oxygen on alveolar macrophage leukotriene B4 synthesis. *Chest, 101*(2), 392–397.

Guyton, A. C., Lindsey, A. W., Abernathy, B., & Richardson, T. (1957). Venous return at various right atrial pressures and the normal venous return curve. *American Journal of Physiology-Legacy Content, 189*(3), 609–615.

Michard, F., & Teboul, J. L. (2002). Predicting fluid responsiveness in ICU patients: a critical analysis of the evidence. *Chest, 121*(6), 2000–2008.

Monnet, X., Marik, P. E., & Teboul, J. L. (2016). Prediction of fluid responsiveness: an update. *Annals of Intensive Care, 6*(1), 1–11.

Sinclair, S. E., Altemeier, W. A., Matute-Bello, G., & Chi, E. Y. (2004). Augmented lung injury due to interaction between hyperoxia and mechanical ventilation. *Critical Care Medicine, 32*(12), 2496–2501.

PART II

ECMO Fundamentals

6

Introduction to ECMO Fundamentals

Let's start our discussion of the fundamentals of extracorporeal membrane oxygenation (ECMO) by returning to our graph. We have spent the last few chapters developing and unpacking the simple but essential concept that the amount of support that is needed for critically ill patients is associated with a dose-related toxicity that increases at higher levels.

The majority of the concept was developed in the context of optimizing oxygen delivery, but the same concept exists for any intervention that is performed in the intensive care unit (ICU). The more sedation, antibiotics, and medications that are needed to support the patient, the greater the potential for drug interactions as well as progressive weakness, delirium, and immobility. It is not simply that sick patients need more support – the support itself can lead to a progressive downward spiral with diminishing positive returns and progressive toxicity that can lead to decompensation and death.

Let's propose now that for specific patients, we can support them with ECMO, a modality that may be associated with some increased risk, but which can hypothetically decrease the degree of dose-related toxicity associated with conventional care (Fig. 6.1).

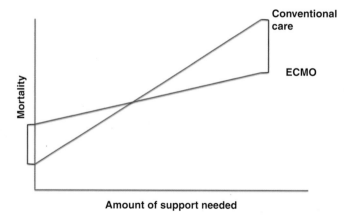

FIG. 6.1 The risk-benefit rationale of ECMO versus conventional care

SO WHAT IS ECMO?

Extracorporeal membrane oxygenation, or ECMO, is a form of extracorporeal life support that functionally involves a blood pump and membrane lung or oxygenator, to support the heart and/or lungs. Let's look at a basic schematic.

The mechanism is deceivingly simple – pumping the blood out of the body, oxygenating the blood, and returning that blood back to the body (Fig. 6.2).

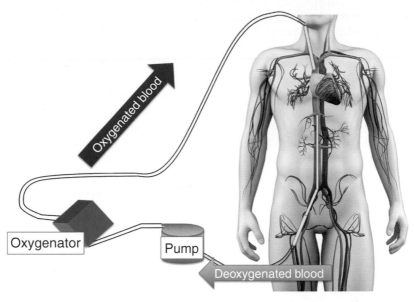

FIG. 6.2 ECMO circuit simplified (Modified from SciePro/Shutterstock.com)

As straightforward as that mechanism is, the physiology of the body that it interacts with can be complex, and forms the basis of the discussions to follow, to truly understand the concepts, physiology, and management principles behind ECMO.

WHY DOES THE ECMO CIRCUIT SEEM MORE COMPLICATED WHEN I LOOK AT IT?

Fig. 6.3 is an example of what might be seen in an ECMO circuit.

It is important to first understand the basics of what ECMO is trying to accomplish. From there, we can fill in the other components that are part of the ECMO circuit. ECMO circuits

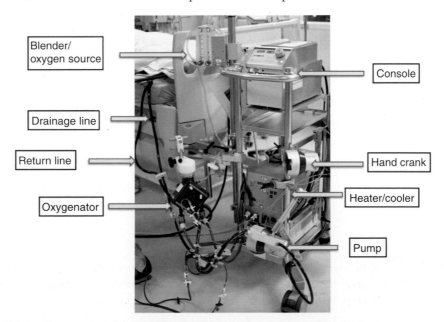

FIG. 6.3 ECMO circuit component (From PIJITRA PHOMKHAM/Shutterstock.com)

have become more straightforward in recent years, but the complexity of the circuit that you are managing can differ widely and is largely determined by institutional protocols, preferences, and processes.

Each component has serves a specific function. Often if this is difficult to distinguish, it can be helpful to trace the circuit in the direction of the blood, reminding ourselves that the basic design is drainage of deoxygenated blood through a pump, through a membrane oxygenator, with the return of oxygenated blood back to the patient.

Let's now better familiarize ourselves with all of the other components, using Fig. 6.4 to help discover various parts of the circuit. We will start in the direction of blood proceeding from the drainage cannula, through the circuit, and finally to the return cannula.

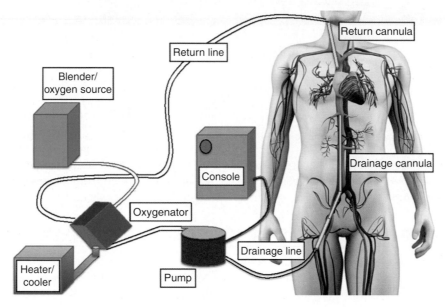

FIG. 6.4 Schematic of ECMO circuit components (Modified from SciePro/Shutterstock.com)

Drainage Cannula

The drainage cannula is the entry point into the ECMO circuit. It is a large-bore access tube that is implanted into the venous circulation through a variety of techniques, including surgical through a graft sewn onto the blood vessel, percutaneously, or through cutdown. It can usually be distinguished from the return cannula in that it is draining dark, deoxygenated blood (Fig. 6.4).

Drainage Line

This is usually a set of clear plastic tubing that is connected to the drainage cannula. The convention is for drainage tubing to be 3/8 of an inch, but this can differ. The drainage line is usually distinguished by the presence of blue tape; however, if this tape is not present, then the color of the blood can be revealing (Fig. 6.4).

Pump

The pump is probably one of the most important components of the ECMO circuit – indeed there is no extracorporeal membrane oxygenation without the ability to circulate blood extracorporeally! However, despite this relative importance of the pump, it can be difficult to notice at first.

If you do not know what you are looking for, then you may miss it. Note the pump, where the blood is entering and where it is exiting. Also at this point, note the backup for the pump, which should always be within arms reach, whether a hand crank, backup console, or backup circuit altogether (Fig. 6.4).

Console

The console is like the dashboard of your car – even though it has nothing to do with actually moving the vehicle forward, it is the interface that you are most likely to interact with. Some consoles can be very straightforward, denoting the speed of the pump and the rate of blood flow only, while others can have a lot of bells and whistles with other data points. The console will usually have some mechanism for altering the revolutions per minute (RPMs), whether a dial or push button (Fig. 6.4).

Oxygenator

The oxygenator is where the membrane oxygenation of ECMO occurs. There are many different types of oxygenator, the common thread being that they have a mechanism for oxygenating the blood through diffusion, and usually a mechanism for temperature regulation (Fig. 6.4).

Blender/Oxygen Source

The oxygenator will be connected to some source of oxygen, usually in the form of a blender, which can be mixed with medical grade air to allow for differing concentrations of oxygen to be delivered. The blender will have the ability to alter the FiO_2 of the gas delivered as well as the rate of the gas flow (known as sweep gas flow). In cases of transport or in emergencies, this oxygen connection can take the form of an oxygen tank, which can deliver 100% FiO_2 at differing sweep gas flow rates (Fig. 6.4).

Heater/Cooler

As we will cover later, the oxygenator is formed by the interface of three phases – blood, oxygen/ sweep gas, and water. The water is used to temperature regulate the blood that is going back to the patient, either warming it to account for ambient loss of temperature in the circuit or cooling it in the case of fever or targeted hypothermia (Fig. 6.4).

Return Line

The return line looks almost identical to the drainage line, with the notable exception that it is filled with oxygenated/bright red blood. The line may also be denoted with red tape, which can be especially important when being connected as a new circuit (Fig. 6.4).

Return Cannula

The destination of the return line is a second cannula that is inserted into the venous or arterial circulation, depending on the type of support being offered. In some cases, the return line can be connected to the return port of a dual lumen cannula that returns blood. We will go into much more detail on the types of drainage/return cannulas when we discuss configurations in Chapter 8.

Overall, that's it! Those are the primary components common to almost every ECMO circuit that you will encounter. There are other components, many of which we will cover in more detail in Chapter 9, but these are the common components that achieve the primary objective of ECMO – drain blood, oxygenate/remove CO_2, temperature regulate, and return the blood to the body. Keep the overall flow straight and you will have a systematic approach to any circuit that you come into contact with.

Now let's go into more detail about what is happening with the fundamental component of ECMO – the oxygenator.

UNDERSTANDING THE OXYGENATOR: THE FUNDAMENTAL MECHANISM OF ECMO

The essence of ECMO is returning oxygenated blood to the body. The oxygenator is where all of this happens. When blood flows through the oxygenator, it enters though an inlet and then follows a specific path, in order to allow for blood to easily pass through while minimizing the entrainment of any air that may come through the circuit (Fig. 6.5).

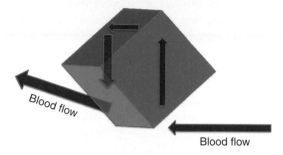

FIG. 6.5 Blood flow through the oxygenator

The oxygenator itself is made of a collection of tiny, hollow plastic tubes that allow for oxygen to flow through. As the blood flows through the oxygenator, it diffuses around the tubes counter-current to the direction of the flow of gas (Fig. 6.6).

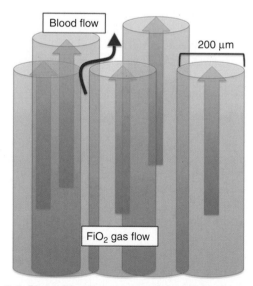

FIG. 6.6 Blood flow through the fibers of the oxygenator

At this level, there is a blood-gas interface, much in the same fashion as what happens at the alveolar level. Just like the alveolar interface, this blood-gas interface allows oxygen to flow down its concentration gradient, from the gas phase in the fibers to the blood, while also allowing CO_2 to go down its concentration gradient, from the blood back into the gas (Fig. 6.7).

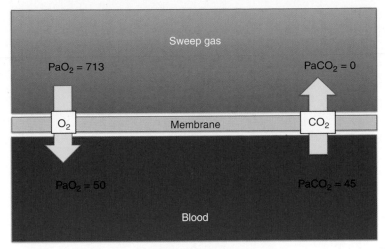

FIG. 6.7 Diffusion of oxygen and carbon dioxide at the membrane level

While all of this is occurring, temperature-controlled water is diffusing around the blood and gas tubules. The water is in a completely separate system – it doesn't come into contact with the blood or sweep gas, but only functions to warm/cool the blood through conduction (Fig. 6.8).

The result is that as blood leaves the oxygenator, it is now oxygenated and temperature controlled, with CO_2 removed. This blood can then be returned to the body.

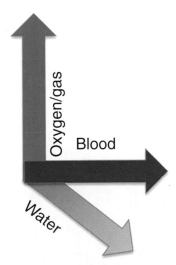

FIG. 6.8 The blood-sweep gas-water interface within the oxygenator

WHERE DOES THE BLOOD GO FROM HERE?

There are two distinct types of ECMO that are defined by where the oxygenated blood is returned. If the blood is drained from the venous side, oxygenated, and returned back into the venous system, it is referred to as veno-venous ECMO, VV ECMO, or sometimes simply respiratory ECMO (Fig. 6.9).

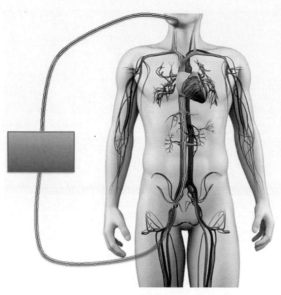

FIG. 6.9 Configurations: veno-venous (VV) (Modified from SciePro/Shutterstock.com)

This configuration allows for oxygenated blood to be returned to the right side of the heart but is dependent on the heart to pump the blood through the circulation. If a significant shunt exists, say due to acute respiratory distress syndrome (ARDS) or pneumonia, the effect of the shunt is reduced because the shunted blood is better oxygenated. If you were not on ECMO, the shunted blood would be shunting from the venous system across the lungs and to the rest of the body.

In contrast, if we were to send the oxygenated blood into the *arterial* system, we now have veno-arterial ECMO, or VA ECMO, or sometimes simply cardiac ECMO (Fig. 6.10).

This configuration allows for oxygenated blood to be returned to the arterial side, so that some/all of the blood is completely bypassing the heart. Any blood that runs through the circuit,

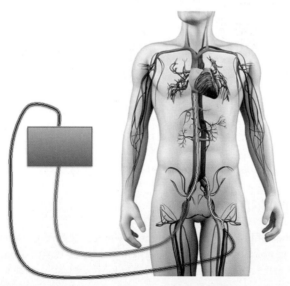

FIG. 6.10 Configurations: veno-arterial (VA) (Modified from SciePro/Shutterstock.com)

therefore, contributes to the perfusion of the body and is *not* dependent on the native cardiac output to do so.

There are many physiologic implications of these two types of support that we will cover in the chapters to come, but for now in the most introductory sense, these are the two primary ways that oxygenated blood can be returned to the body.

HOW CAN I MANIPULATE THE CIRCUIT?

There are really only a couple of mechanisms that can be manipulated on an ECMO machine:
1. RPMs/blood flow
2. Sweep gas flow
3. Temperature
   That's it. Let's review.

Revolutions Per Minute

Altering the RPM is one of the most fundamental changes that can be done to the circuit. Increasing the RPMs increases the speed that the centrifugal pump turns and, consequently, can induce higher blood flow. There are many factors that affect how RPMs correlate with flow, which we will cover in greater detail when we discuss flow physiology in Chapter 10.

For the present time, suffice it to say that an increase in RPMs is analogous to a motor in a car – the faster the motor turns, the faster the car goes.

RPMs are usually manipulated on the console, whether in the form of a dial or a button. There will also be a display on the console that will denote the number of RPMs that the pump is currently running at as well as the consequent blood flow (Fig. 6.11).

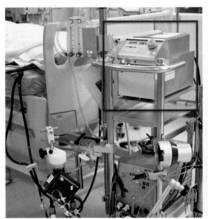 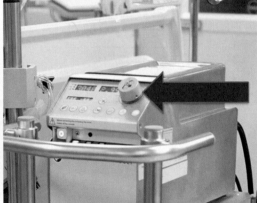

FIG. 6.11 ECMO settings: revolutions per minute/flow (From PIJITRA PHOMKHAM/Shutterstock.com)

Sweep Gas Flow/FiO$_2$

Sweep gas is the gas that is infused into the membrane. There are two fundamental changes that can be made to it – the rate of gas flow and the FiO$_2$ of this gas (Fig. 6.12).

Usually the manipulations are made to the blender as denoted earlier. In this case, the knob on the far right allows for changes in FiO$_2$, from 21% (room air) to 100% FiO$_2$.

The sweep gas flow rates are adjusted with the knob to the left of the FiO$_2$ knob, going from 0 to 10 L/min. The knob to the far left is for smaller increments of the final liter of flow from

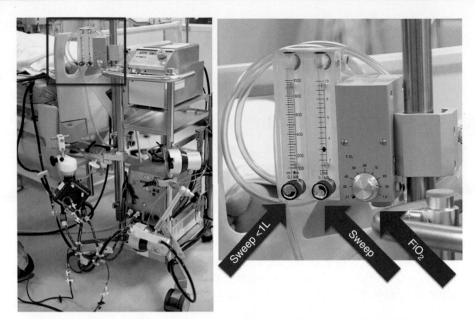

FIG. 6.12 ECMO settings: sweep gas flow/FiO$_2$ (From PIJITRA PHOMKHAM/Shutterstock.com)

0 to 1000 mL (1 L) per minute. Note that any flow on this knob is in addition to the flow demarcated in the middle knob.

What Are the Effects of Manipulations to Sweep Gas Flow and ECMO Blood Flow to the Patient?

We will go into this in much more detail in the ECMO Physiology section, but for now, the basic direction is as follows:

> FiO$_2$ and ECMO blood flow affect **oxygenation/oxygen delivery** while sweep gas flow affects **ventilation/CO$_2$ removal**

Temperature

The final setting that can be adjusted on the ECMO circuit is the temperature of the blood that is returned to the body. This adjustment is made much less frequently than blood flow or sweep gas flow/FiO$_2$. That said, this mechanism allows for the close maintenance of temperature, even to the tenth of a degree (Fig. 6.13).

PUTTING IT ALL TOGETHER

We went over a lot in this chapter in order to give a very high-level overview of ECMO – to include the rationale behind the use of ECMO, how the ECMO circuit works, introduction to the components, configurations, and, finally, how the circuit can be manipulated.

Hopefully you will agree that the rationale and mechanism behind ECMO is relatively straightforward. This does not mean the management of ECMO itself is straightforward. Instead, as we will continue to appreciate, the complexity arises from the physiology with which the ECMO circuit interacts. However, we will continue to develop a systematic approach to the

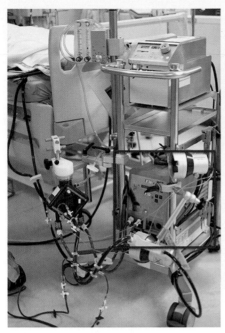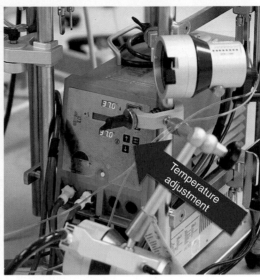

FIG. 6.13 ECMO settings: temperature (From PIJITRA PHOMKHAM/Shutterstock.com)

various aspects of the ECMO circuit, including its physiology, in order to build confidence and understanding of the concepts related to ECMO.

But we are just getting started. We will continue to develop this approach in the next chapter when we take on how we can approach selecting patients for ECMO.

SUGGESTED READING

Brodie, D., & Bacchetta, M. (2011). Extracorporeal membrane oxygenation for ARDS in adults. *New England Journal of Medicine, 365*(20), 1905–1914.

Lehle, K., Philipp, A., Gleich, O., Holzamer, A., Müller, T., & Bein, T., et al. (2008). Efficiency in extracorporeal membrane oxygenation—cellular deposits on polymethypentene membranes increase resistance to blood flow and reduce gas exchange capacity. *ASAIO Journal, 54*(6), 612–617.

Lequier, L., Horton, S. B., McMullan, D. M., & Bartlett, R. H. (2013). Extracorporeal membrane oxygenation circuitry. *Pediatric Critical Care Medicine: A Journal of the Society of Critical Care Medicine and the World Federation of Pediatric Intensive and Critical Care Societies, 14*(5 Suppl 1), S7.

Lim, M. W. (2006). The history of extracorporeal oxygenators. *Anaesthesia, 61*(10), 984–995.

7

Indications and Selection of Patients for ECMO

In this chapter, we tackle one of the most sobering and important topics related to extracorporeal membrane oxygenation (ECMO) – selection of patients for ECMO. In doing so, we are trying to reconcile two very important and weighty decisions:

1. Can I choose someone for ECMO who would be likely to do well with ECMO?
2. Can I spare someone the risks of ECMO if they are unlikely to benefit?

These can be challenging to parse out and can weigh heavily on clinicians. To better understand this dynamic, let's return to our graph comparing ECMO to conventional care (Fig. 7.1).

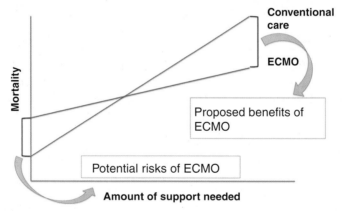

FIG. 7.1 Proposed risks and benefits of ECMO versus conventional care

The green line (ECMO) starts out the graph significantly higher than the blue line (conventional care), which represents that ECMO has a cost in terms of risk. Simply cannulating means inserting large cannulas into major blood vessels leading to all of the associated risks – pseudoaneurisms, damage to underlying structures, extremity ischemia, dissection, etc. Even if your team is excellent at cannulating with very few complications, you are exposing blood to foreign surfaces and altering the coagulation cascade, which could alter bleeding and hemodynamics down the road. Even from a resource standpoint, putting someone on ECMO can be expensive and resource intensive.

Given all this, you may be asking yourself some hard questions.

"Aren't people either not sick enough to even consider ECMO or so sick that ECMO would not be of benefit?"

Or even more so, "Why even put someone on ECMO?"

These questions get to the heart of the challenge of selection for ECMO. While challenging, there is a sweet spot that exists – teams that are truly adept at selection are able to identify that select group of patients that is likely to do poorly without ECMO and will improve with ECMO (Fig. 7.2). This is the art of selection, which we will spend this entire chapter trying to refine.

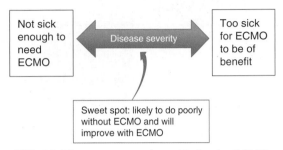

FIG. 7.2 The sweet spot for selection for ECMO

SO HOW CAN WE GET BETTER AT FINDING THIS SELECT GROUP OF PATIENTS?

To tease out this select patient population, let's consider the following rules, to help us hit that sweet spot with regards to selection for ECMO.

> Rule 1: **Reversible** etiology of cardiac or respiratory failure
> Rule 2: Conventional therapy is harming the patient more than helping
> Rule 3: Cardiac/respiratory failure has to be severe enough to justify the risks of ECMO
> Rule 4: Patient is not too far gone so that ECMO will not be of benefit

Let's explore a little more of what is behind each rule.

Rule 1: Reversible Etiology of Cardiac or Respiratory Failure

This is an essential rule and an acknowledgement that ECMO does little to fix the underlying disorder. Rather, a path must exist towards eventual recovery or destination (such as a transplant, long-term device, etc.).

Often, while recovery can exist, there is some barrier that is preventing this, whether it is the high ventilator requirements or escalating pressors. What the patient needs is time to allow for eventual recovery. This time is what ECMO can offer (Fig. 7.3).

The reversibility of the underlying cause of severe respiratory/cardiac failure will be a strong factor in a patient's candidacy for ECMO. Ideally, the more readily reversible the condition, the better, especially if the risk of decompensation without ECMO is significant. A patient with severe, refractory status asthmaticus, with an anticipated recovery of 24–48 hours on ECMO, has very different risk profile from a patient with ARDS from bacterial pneumonia, who may have an anticipated recovery of weeks to months. Likewise, a patient with a normal heart and cardiogenic shock from a pulmonary embolism may carry a very different risk profile from a patient with chronic cardiomyopathy and decompensated heart failure.

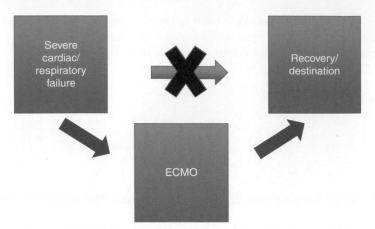

FIG. 7.3 The role of ECMO in arriving at recovery/destination in reversible conditions

Rule 2: Conventional Therapy Is Harming the Patient More Than Helping

We spent a great deal of time in Part 1 defining and outlining the dose-related toxicity of conventional care. All the things that can be done in the intensive care unit (ICU) to optimize oxygen delivery (pressors, inotropes, oxygen, positive pressure ventilation, fluid, blood) come with a cost that compounds with increasing dose.

These interventions combine diminishing returns with increased toxicity at higher levels. This means that the higher the dose of conventional supportive care is not only needed for sicker patients, but actually that conventional supportive care itself can be harmful at higher doses.

ECMO has to spare some degree of this toxicity. The more toxicity that can be potentially spared, the stronger the rationale for ECMO.

Rule 3: Cardiac/Respiratory Failure Has to Be Severe Enough to Justify the Risks of ECMO

It is one thing to say that conventional therapy is harming the patient more than helping. It is quite another to say that the degree that it is harming the patient is severe enough that sparing this harm is worth the risks of placing a patient on ECMO.

Let's suppose for example that you have a patient on a ventilator for pneumonia. The ventilator is set at 100% FiO_2, and he has been on this oxygen level for days.

Is there toxicity associated with this level of support? Certainly.

Does this toxicity justify the risks of ECMO? Maybe not.

To answer this question, we would need to really understand how dependent the patient was on this high level of support and what trajectory the patient was on. Otherwise, our graph may look something like Fig. 7.4, with the conventional support line increasing from left to right but not increasing to the degree that it would intersect with the ECMO line.

How can we quantify the response to the level of support and the trajectory? Let's consider a few parameters.

Respiratory Thresholds of Severity

Let's return to our patient with pneumonia. He may be on a harmful amount of oxygen with the ventilator set at 100%, but the true severity of his respiratory failure will be determined by his response to the high level of support. We can define this response by looking at the function of the lungs: to oxygenate (provide O_2) and to ventilate (remove CO_2). Remember that both of these functions can be performed, because these gases are able to flow down their relative concentration gradients at the level of the blood-alveolar interface (Fig. 7.5).

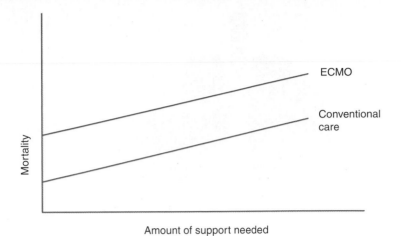

FIG. 7.4 The limited benefits of ECMO over conventional care in the case of lower disease severity

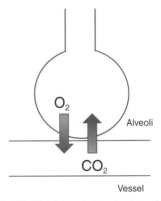

FIG. 7.5 The blood-alveolar interface

The oxygen that diffuses across the lungs is dissolved into the blood until it saturates the hemoglobin and can be efficiently delivered to the tissues. The amount of oxygen that is dissolved in the blood, or the PaO_2, will give an indicator of how well the lungs are oxygenating – the worse the lungs are performing, the lower the PaO_2.

A PaO_2 of 60 mmHg on room air (21% FiO_2) represents a very different clinical situation than a PaO_2 of 60 mmHg on 100% FiO_2, as you would expect a much higher PaO_2 if you were administering 100% FiO_2. The convention for quantifying this is to express the PaO_2 as a ratio to the FiO_2, otherwise known as a PaO_2:FiO_2 ratio, or a P:F. As shunt increases, we have worsening P:F ratio that is less responsive to increases in FiO_2. To combat this, we will have to increase alveolar recruitment through raising the mean airway pressure (Fig. 7.6).

Remember also that as lungs become progressively more compromised, compliance also decreases and it takes more pressure from the ventilator to obtain the same tidal volume with each breath (Fig. 7.7).

This can also contribute to a worsening ventilatory function of the lungs. When we are unable to adequately oxygenate/remove CO_2 despite optimal management of the ventilator, we can

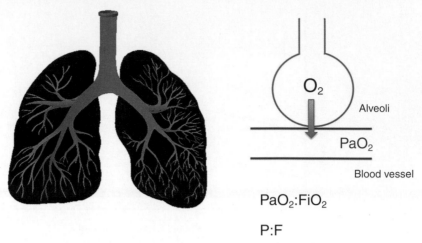

FIG. 7.6 The PaO_2 to FiO_2 ratio in respiratory failure. (Modified from YanGe_Tam/Shutterstock.com.)

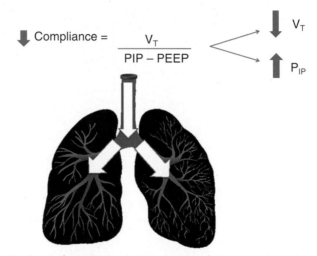

FIG. 7.7 The limitations of ventilation in the setting of decreased respiratory compliance. *VT*, tidal volume, *PIP*, inspiratory pressure, *PEEP*, positive end expiratory pressure. (Modified from YanGe_Tam/Shutterstock.com.)

consider ECMO. This threshold is not well defined, but a reasonable starting point for discussion is a failure of oxygenation with **P:F < 100** or a failure of ventilation with respiratory acidosis and a **pH < 7.25** despite optimal mechanical ventilation.

Cardiac Thresholds of Severity

Cardiac thresholds for considering ECMO are not always as well defined, but they should be carefully considered.

In a similar fashion to our discussion of respiratory failure, the maintenance of cardiac output is essential for two tasks: maintenance of the vascular pressure head through generation of adequate mean arterial pressure and perfusion of end organs. Doing one without the other is insufficient for delivering oxygen and upkeep of metabolic function. Therefore, the evaluation for thresholds of cardiac failure should involve an evaluation of both the mean arterial pressure and the perfusion of end organs. Thus, let's examine the following parameters for consideration of VA ECMO (Fig. 7.8).

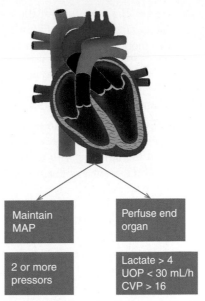

FIG. 7.8 Thresholds of cardiac failure in cardiogenic shock. (Modified from Ody_Stocker/Shutterstock.com.). *CVP*, Central venous pressure; *MAP*, mean arterial pressure; *UOP*, Urine output.

Selection for VA ECMO should also include consideration of the physiology and nature of the insult and placed in the context of other forms of mechanical circulatory support (i.e., whether an intraaortic balloon pump/percutaneous ventricular assist device be a better form of support for the patient given their physiology). We will discuss this in much greater detail in the VA ECMO physiology sections.

Urgency for Consideration of ECMO

As a final note, these parameters should be put into the context of the clinical trajectory and urgency for consideration of ECMO. To return to our graphs, the intersection of the two lines would be considered the threshold for initiating ECMO (Fig. 7.9A). Therefore, in a situation where the patient is severely decompensated, like on the graph on the right, there would be a much lower threshold of consideration for ECMO (Fig. 7.9B).

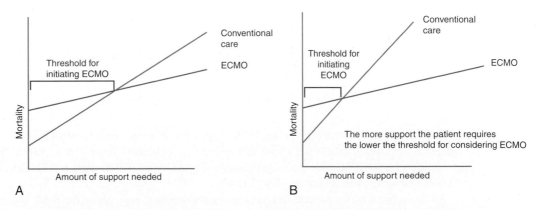

FIG. 7.9 Lower threshold for initiating ECMO in the case of higher disease severity

The worse the parameters, the more urgent the consideration for ECMO. For example, for two patients with respiratory failure with the following gases, Patient A might signal a failure to oxygenate/ventilate, with a more urgent consideration for ECMO:

Patient A: 7.15, $PaCO_2$ 75, PaO_2 40 on 100%

Patient B: 7.35, $PaCO_2$ 50, PaO_2 85 on 100% FiO_2

Rule 4: Patient Is Not Too Far Gone So That ECMO Will Not Be of Benefit

If you are going to offer ECMO, you want to make sure that it is of benefit. You do not want to offer it to someone who does not have a reversible condition and may never get better, nor would you want to offer it to someone who does not have some toxicity that you can spare them. Likewise, you would not want to offer it to someone who is not sick enough to justify the risks of initiating support.

In a similar fashion, you must carefully evaluate patients, especially sicker patients, for being so decompensated that ECMO will not be beneficial. This can include patients in multi-organ failure, patients with prolonged CPR, prolonged periods on mechanical ventilation, increasing age/comorbidities, and irreversible malignancies with a limited lifespan.

Sometimes, it can be relatively straightforward to deduce that initiation of ECMO is not worth the risks to the patient. Sometimes, it can be difficult to pick the time when the patient is in a nonrecoverable state, especially as you consider the case of escalating disease severity.

As illustrated in Fig. 7.10, the more decompensated a patient with cardiac/respiratory failure, the more likely they will benefit from ECMO, until a point when there is evidence of irreversible damage, and then the benefit rapidly becomes less apparent.

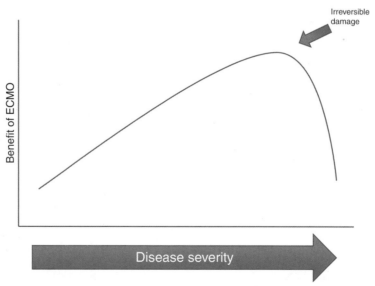

FIG. 7.10 Disease severity and the potential benefit of ECMO

What defines "irreversible damage"? This can be a difficult point to recognize. Is it a lactate cutoff in cardiogenic shock? Is it a specific time on the ventilator? You will find that the longer you evaluate patients for ECMO, the more nuanced of a sense you will develop for which patients will do well and which will do poorly (Fig. 7.11A).

To finish our analogy, patients too decompensated are like the graph on the right, where the slope of the conventional care line is so steep that it does not even intersect with the ECMO line (Fig. 7.11B).

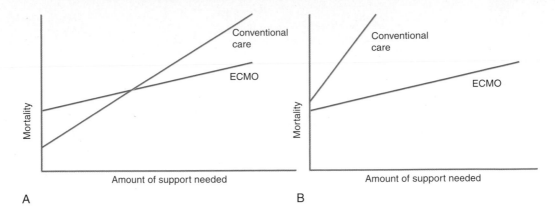

FIG. 7.11 Limited benefit of ECMO in the setting of irreversible damage

PUTTING IT ALL TOGETHER

When it comes to selecting for ECMO, I think intent is paramount. The four rules presented in this chapter are to help define that important population of patients that would benefit from ECMO who would likely do poorly without ECMO. They are not to make numbers and mortality look better. When we are considering whether we should initiate support, we need to define and quantify the gap between outcomes with and without ECMO and weigh that gap against the ability to provide that care. A large ECMO program performing its 200th ECMO run may be more willing to take on a more complex patient than a program with less experience, resources, and capabilities.

At the end of the day, selecting patients for ECMO requires great humility and a realization of the limits of our knowledge and predicting capability. Although we may be not able to predict the overall outcome with absolute certainty, if we are approaching every evaluation with the desire to find patients who are likely to derive benefit while eliminating the consideration of patients who are likely to derive harm, we are certainly on the right path.

SUGGESTED READING

Combes, A., Hajage, D., Capellier, G., Demoule, A., Lavoué, S., & Guervilly, C., et al. (2018). Extracorporeal membrane oxygenation for severe acute respiratory distress syndrome. *New England Journal of Medicine, 378*(21), 1965–1975.

Enger, T., Philipp, A., Videm, V., Lubnow, M., Wahba, A., & Fischer, M., et al. (2014). Prediction of mortality in adult patients with severe acute lung failure receiving veno-venous extracorporeal membrane oxygenation: a prospective observational study. *Critical Care, 18*(2), 1–10.

Peek, G. J., Mugford, M., Tiruvoipati, R., Wilson, A., Allen, E., & Thalanany, M. M., et al. (2009). Efficacy and economic assessment of conventional ventilatory support versus extracorporeal membrane oxygenation for severe adult respiratory failure (CESAR): a multicentre randomised controlled trial. *The Lancet, 374*(9698), 1351–1363.

Schmidt, M., Zogheib, E., Rozé, H., Repesse, X., Lebreton, G., & Luyt, C. E., et al. (2013). The PRESERVE mortality risk score and analysis of long-term outcomes after extracorporeal membrane oxygenation for severe acute respiratory distress syndrome. *Intensive Care Medicine, 39*, 1704–1713.

Schmidt, M., et al. (2015). Predicting survival after ECMO for refractory cardiogenic shock: the survival after veno-arterial-ECMO (SAVE)-score. *European Heart Journal, 36*(33), 2246–2256.

8

ECMO Configurations

Let's now continue our exploration of the fundamentals of extracorporeal membrane oxygenation (ECMO) support by discussing cannulation configurations. To remind ourselves, the basic function of the ECMO circuit is to drain deoxygenated blood, remove CO_2/oxygenate in the membrane oxygenator, and return that blood back to the body (Fig. 8.1).

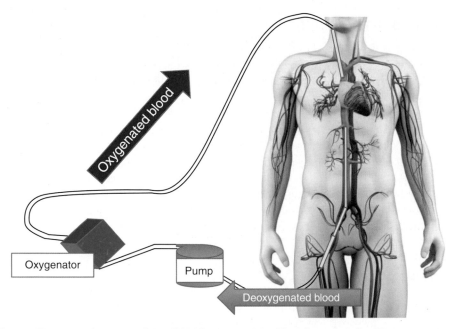

FIG. 8.1 The basic function of the ECMO circuit. (Modified from SciePro/Shutterstock.com.)

Where this blood is drained from and where it returns to is exactly what we will go over in this chapter. We will cover a lot of configuration possibilities and when possible, the relevant physiologic rationale. This chapter is neither a comprehensive compilation, nor is every configuration mentioned used by every cannulating team, as some may be related to the preferences of the team. If anything, the breadth of this list underscores the many possibilities that exist for configuring the ECMO circuit to the specific physiologic needs of the patient.

CANNULA SELECTION

The first consideration is size and type of cannulas. Cannulas are large catheters that are inserted into heart or blood vessels by which blood is drained and returned. Most of the time, one cannula drains the blood while the other cannula returns the blood. These two cannulas often differ by where holes are placed for drainage and return of blood. There are primarily two types of cannulas that should be distinguished, referred to as multistage and single stage (Fig. 8.2).

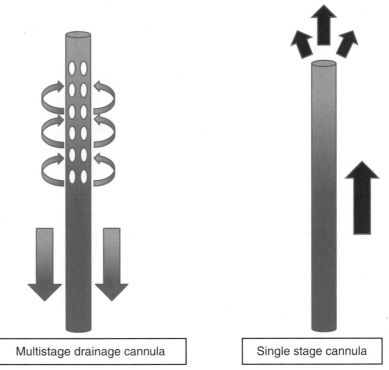

Multistage drainage cannula

Single stage cannula

FIG. 8.2 Multistage drainage cannula (left) with multiple drainage holes and singe stage cannula (right) with single point of exit for blood

Multistage cannulas are usually used as the drainage cannula. When draining blood, you want to have the ability to pull in blood over a large surface area so that a sufficient volume of blood can be run through the circuit without excessive negative pressure to do so. Thus, multistage cannulas have multiple holes for draining blood.

Compare this to the single-stage cannula, which has only one set of holes at the top. This carries the advantage of allowing for directional flow of returned blood. The single-stage return cannula can differ in length, usually being around 15 cm for short return cannulas and 50 cm for long return cannulas.

The other type of cannula is the dual lumen cannula. Dual lumen cannulas embed a return cannula inside an outer, drainage cannula as illustrated in Fig. 8.3. There is an outlet that allows for the return of oxygenated blood that can be aimed in a manner so that it does not get pulled back into the ECMO circuit. Dual lumen cannulas allow for both drainage and return of blood from a single access site, which can allow for improved mobility and ambulation.

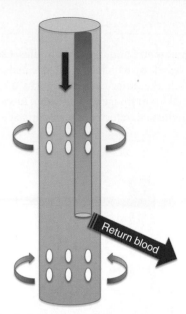

FIG. 8.3 Dual lumen cannula draining blood from outer lumen and returning blood through inner lumen

The final consideration for cannula selection is width and length. The length can vary but for the most part is fairly standard for multistage cannulas, all being around 50 cm for adults. The length of the return cannula depends on where the cannula is being implanted and for the most part remains as a long return (~50 cm) or a short return (~15 cm) (Fig. 8.4).

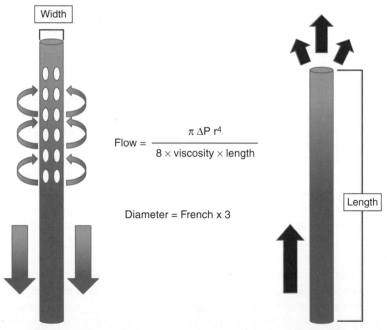

$$\text{Flow} = \frac{\pi \, \Delta P \, r^4}{8 \times \text{viscosity} \times \text{length}}$$

$$\text{Diameter} = \text{French} \times 3$$

FIG. 8.4 Width and length considerations in cannula selection

Width is an important consideration for cannula selection, as the width is an important determination of overall flow – the wider the cannula, the more flow you will be able to obtain. We will talk about the concept of flow in much greater detail in Chapter 10. The benefits of greater flow have to be weighed against the possibility of greater obstruction of the blood vessel, more damage to the blood vessels, and whether or not the vessels can accommodate a larger cannula.

The standard convention for width is French, which is three times the diameter of the cannula in millimeters. This can be helpful when sizing cannulas to the size of the blood vessel. If the blood vessel is 6 mm, for example, then it likely could not accommodate a 21-French cannula, which would have a diameter of 7 mm.

NAMING CONVENTION

First off, let's review the basic naming convention. Typically, the name of the configuration follows the direction of blood. If you are draining blood from the venous system and returning it to the arterial system, then this is referred to as **Veno-Arterial ECMO** or **VA** ECMO (Fig. 8.5).

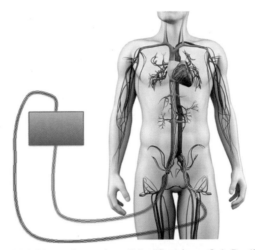

FIG. 8.5 Veno-arterial (VA) configuration. (Modified from SciePro/Shutterstock.com.)

Contrast this to the following configuration, where we are draining from the venous system and returning back to the venous system. This is referred to as **Veno-Venous ECMO**, or **VV** ECMO (Fig. 8.6).

Now let's look at some configurations, starting with VV ECMO.

FEMORAL JUGULAR VV ECMO

Femoral-jugular involves a drainage cannula that is implanted into the inferior vena cava (IVC) via the common femoral vein and a short return cannula implanted into the superior vena cava (SVC)/right atrial junction via the internal jugular vein (Fig. 8.7). The drainage cannula is usually a multistage cannula to allow for optimal drainage and positioning. Ideally, the drainage cannula should be inserted into the intrahepatic IVC right under the diaphragm. The intrahepatic IVC position allows for the liver parenchyma to keep the IVC open and helps to optimize flow without collapse of the IVC around the negative pressure generated from the drainage ports.

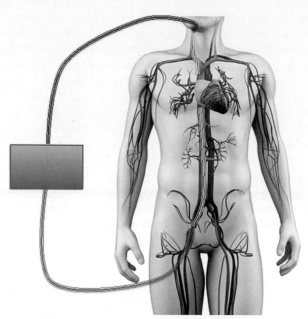

FIG. 8.6 Veno-venous (VV) configuration. (Modified from SciePro/Shutterstock.com.)

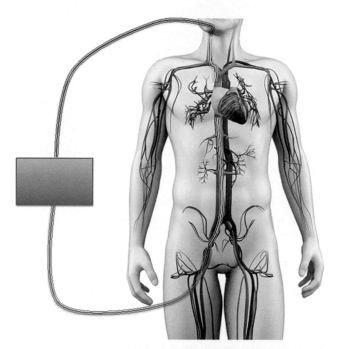

FIG. 8.7 Femoral jugular configuration. (Modified from SciePro/Shutterstock.com.)

The return cannula, by contrast, should be a short, single-stage cannula, implanted into the right or left internal jugular vein, although the right IJ vein allows a somewhat straighter path to the optimal position in the RA/SVC junction. Placing the return cannula in the SVC/RA junction, with the drainage cannula lower at the intrahepatic IVC just below the diaphragm, separates the two cannulas and prevents oxygenated blood that is being returned from the ECMO circuit to be sucked back into the circuit, a concept known as recirculation, which we will cover in more detail later on.

FEMORAL-FEMORAL VV ECMO

Femoral-femoral VV ECMO involves a multistage drainage cannula placed into the intrahepatic IVC just like in the femoral-IJ configuration; however, in this configuration, the return cannula is a long, single-stage cannula implanted into the IVC/RA junction from below, via that contra-lateral femoral vein (Fig. 8.8). Since the return cannula is a single-stage cannula, and is inserted above the top of the drainage cannula, blood can theoretically be returned without being sucked back into the drainage cannula in the form of recirculation. However, this risk of recirculation can be more significant with this configuration than with femoral-jugular.

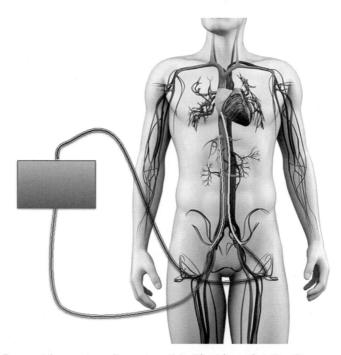

FIG. 8.8 Femoral-femoral configuration. (Modified from SciePro/Shutterstock.com.)

ADDITIONAL VENOUS DRAIN

Intermittently, you may come across a circuit with two drainage cannulas. To confirm it is two drainage cannulas as opposed to two return cannulas, ensure that both cannulas are draining dark blood.

What is the advantage of an additional drainage cannula? Some providers use a second cannula if obtaining adequate flows are insufficient. Usually, if a second cannula is added for improved flow, it is a drainage cannula, as the flow limitations on VV ECMO are often dictated by the drainage side (Fig. 8.9).

This is a configuration that is rarely used, simply because a properly sized drainage cannula, placed into good position in the intrahepatic IVC, is often able to obtain more than adequate flows. However, there are rare instances (for example, in the development of abdominal compartment syndrome due to bleeding) where even a well-positioned drain cannula cannot obtain

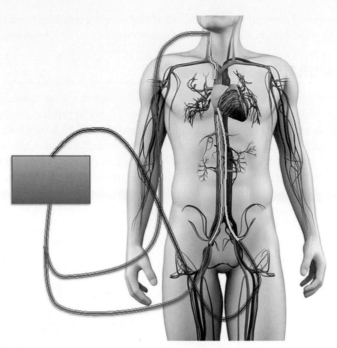

FIG. 8.9 Additional venous drain. (Modified from SciePro/Shutterstock.com.)

the adequate flows. In this case, an additional drain cannula may be added and connected to the circuit through a Y-connection (Fig. 8.23B).

DUAL LUMEN CANNULA

The dual lumen cannula offers the ability to drain blood from the outer cannula with an inner cannula, which can return blood. In the standard cannula configuration, this is inserted in the intrahepatic IVC via the right internal jugular vein, which carries the benefit of being the straightest path. In the proper configuration, the outlet port lines up with the right atrium with the outflow track flowing across the tricuspid valve, with inlet ports positioned above and below the outlet ports (Fig. 8.10).

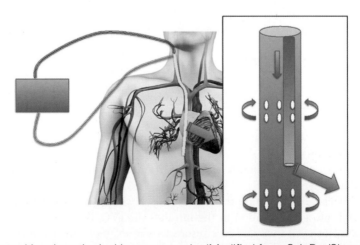

FIG. 8.10 Internal jugular vein dual lumen cannula. (Modified from SciePro/Shutterstock.com.)

Dual Lumen Cannula in Subclavian Position

As compared to the IJ approach, the subclavian approach can be more stable, with less rotation and better positioning of the outflow track across the tricuspid valve. Consequently, this configuration can better facilitate mobility, with less worry about rotational positioning. However, this configuration can be more technically challenging to implant (Fig. 8.11).

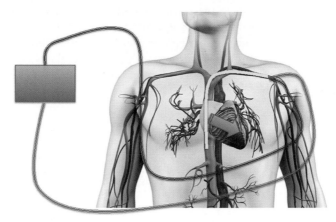

FIG. 8.11 Subclavian vein dual lumen cannula. (Modified from SciePro/Shutterstock.com.)

Dual Lumen IJ-PA Configuration

A different dual lumen cannula offers the ability to drain from the SVC/right atrium and return blood directly into the pulmonary artery. This is accomplished by implanting the cannula from the IJ vein into the SVC/right atrium, across the tricuspid valve into the right ventricle, and across the pulmonic valve into the pulmonary artery, as illustrated in Fig. 8.12.

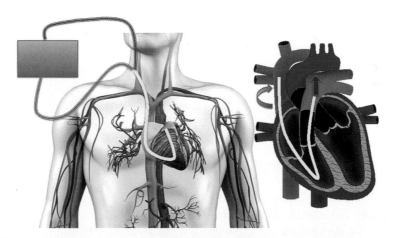

FIG. 8.12 Dual lumen IJ-PA cannula. (Modified from SciePro/Shutterstock.com and Ody_Stocker/Shutterstock.com.)

This configuration requires a slightly different cannula, which is longer to reach all the way to the pulmonary artery that has the outflow track at the tip of the cannula instead of out the side.

This configuration carries the benefit of draining blood from the right ventricle and returning blood past the pulmonic valve, so it provides oxygenated blood in addition to providing some right heart support. Additionally, there is theoretically less chance of recirculation as the pulmonic valve separates the inflow holes from the outflow track. However, this cannula can be more technically challenging to implant and manage.

FEMORAL-PA VV ECMO

If a dual lumen cannula to reach the pulmonary artery is not available or preferred, a similar configuration can be obtained by draining from the IVC via a multistage cannula implanted into the femoral vein and returning into the pulmonary artery via a long, single-stage, cannula implanted into the pulmonary artery via the IJ vein. This configuration would still provide VV ECMO support and right ventricular support but would require two-site cannulation (Fig. 8.13).

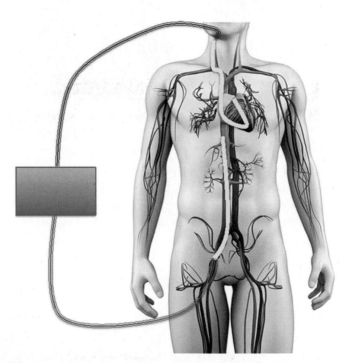

FIG. 8.13 Femoral-PA cannula. (Modified from SciePro/Shutterstock.com.)

VA ECMO: FEMORAL-FEMORAL

Percutaneously placed VA ECMO tends to be much more straightforward than VV ECMO. For adults, the near universal configuration is a multistage cannula implanted in the intrahepatic IVC via the femoral vein and a short, single-stage return cannula implanted into the distal aorta via the femoral artery (Fig. 8.14).

The arterial cannula directs blood retrograde towards the heart. Consequently, a short cannula works the best for this function, as a longer cannula would bypass much of the splanchnic and renal blood supply. We will go over the physiology related to this retrograde flow in much more detail in Chapter 14.

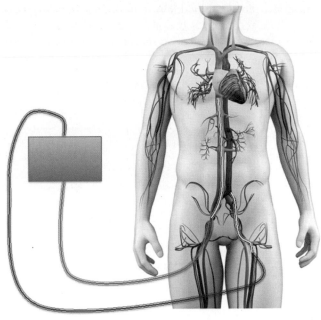

FIG. 8.14 Femoral-femoral VA ECMO configuration. (Modified from SciePro/Shutterstock.com.)

ARTERIAL ACCESS FOR VA ECMO

Placement of an arterial cannula carries the unique challenge of the cannula impeding forward, arterial flow to the distal, ipsilateral extremity (Fig. 8.15).

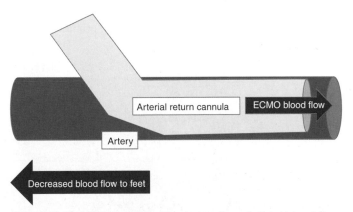

FIG. 8.15 Arterial cannula with obstruction of distal blood flow

There are a few strategies to mitigate this adverse effect:
1. Placement of a small enough cannula to allow for forward blood flow around the cannula
2. Placement of a graft on the artery to allow for flow both retrograde towards the aorta and ante-grade down the leg
3. Placement of a distal perfusion cannula into the superficial femoral artery with diversion of oxygenated blood from the return line down the leg for better perfusion

Arterial grafts allow for blood flow in both directions but require a surgical cutdown and can have some technical considerations, as the angle of the graft can determine the amount of blood flow in either direction, potentially resulting in overflow/underflow (Fig. 8.16).

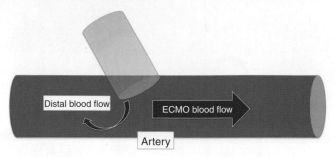

FIG. 8.16 Arterial graft with bidirectional blood flow

The distal perfusion catheter can potentially be placed percutaneously and can allow for blood flow directly from the ECMO circuit (Fig. 8.17).

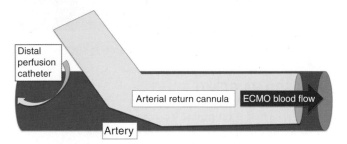

FIG. 8.17 Arterial cannula with distal perfusion catheter

The sheath can become occluded or kinked, so should be flushed intermittently (Fig. 8.18).

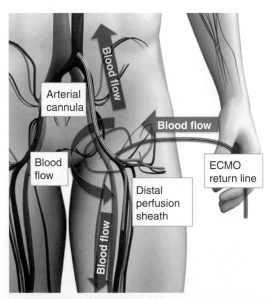

FIG. 8.18 Connection of distal perfusion catheter to return limb of the ECMO circuit (Modified from SciePro/Shutterstock.com.)

VA ECMO: SURGICAL CANNULATION

Surgical access for VA ECMO allows for other configurations. The first is the standard graft that can be sewn on the artery, allowing for access to either the femoral artery or access to smaller vessels like the axillary artery (Fig. 8.19).

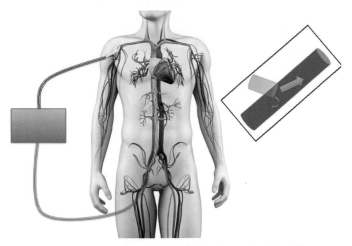

FIG. 8.19 VA ECMO with axillary graft. (Modified from SciePro/Shutterstock.com.)

The axillary artery graft allows for more mobility as there is no limitation of a femoral arterial cannula. Additionally, it carries the added advantage of allowing for antegrade flow. There are technical challenges including the need to obtain the right angle, lest the arm gets too much or two little blood.

IJ AXILLARY CANNULATION

Other models can be employed to allow for complete upper body cannulation, for example, the IJ-axillary cannulation. This can further facilitate mobility (Fig. 8.20).

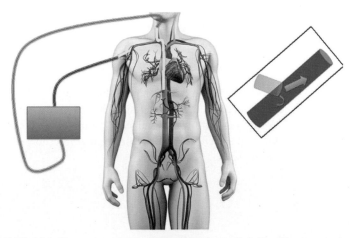

FIG. 8.20 IJ axillary cannulation. (Modified from SciePro/Shutterstock.com.)

CENTRAL CANNULATION: FEMORAL AORTIC

If any cannulas/grafts are implanted directly into the heart or great vessels, this is often referred to as central cannulation. The return cannula is implanted into a graft sewn directly onto the aorta, which allows for antegrade flow. Since the chest is often open when cannulating in this manner, this is frequently combined with a drain in the left ventricle, which allows for the direct removal of blood, mitigating left ventricular distension in a process called venting. We will discuss this configuration in much more detail in Chapter 15.

The drainage in these cases can either be a femoral drain, which is often implanted percutaneously, or a graft that is sewn directly onto the right atrium (Figs. 8.21 and 8.22).

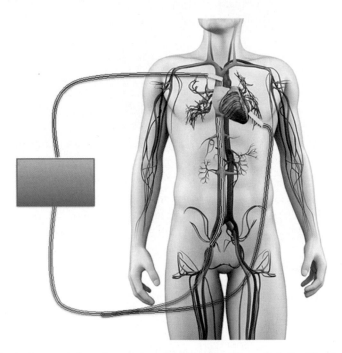

FIG. 8.21 Central cannulation: femoral-aortic. (Modified from SciePro/Shutterstock.com.)

While there can be advantages to this cannulation strategy, often the chest is left open, which can have many ancillary effects to include risk of infection, inability to wean sedation/analgesic, immobility, and requirement of mechanical ventilation. In some cases, the cannulas can be tunneled out of the skin and the chest can be closed. However, there will exist the need for eventual return to the Operating room (OR) for removal.

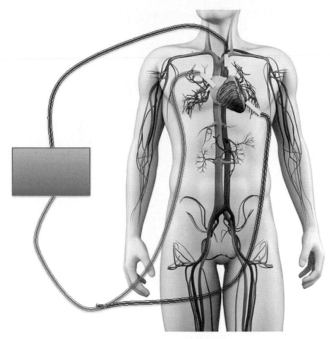

FIG. 8.22 Centgral cannulation: RA-aortic with left ventricular drain (Modified from SciePro/Shutterstock.com.)

HYBRID CONFIGURATIONS: WHERE VA AND VV MEET

Intermittently, additional cannulas can be added to a VV/VA circuit, in order to form a hybrid configuration. These cannulas drain blood that is connected through a Y connector that can direct the flow of blood in two directions as illustrated in Fig. 8.23A,B.

This is where naming convention is important as it is easy to confuse how blood is flowing. Remember, the configuration is named in the direction of blood. If you are Y connecting two venous drains while maintaining one arterial return, then this is called VVA, as illustrated in Fig. 8.24A,B.

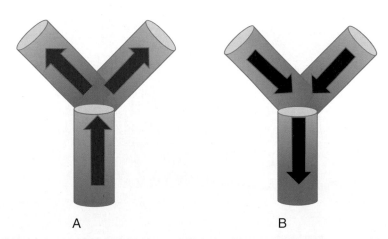

A   B

FIG. 8.23 A: Y connection for returned blood. B: Y connection for drained blood

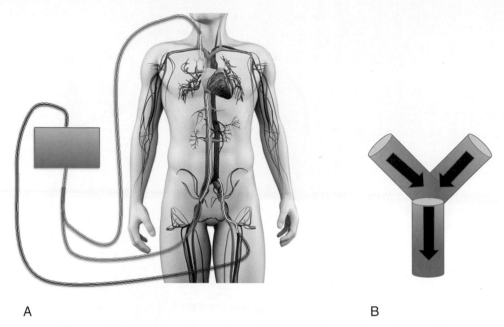

FIG. 8.24 VVA hybrid configuration with Y connection on the drainage side (Modified from SciePro/Shutterstock.com.)

Compare this to the more common hybrid configuration, where the return line is split between returning to an arterial and a venous cannula. This would be named as VAV ECMO, as illustrated in Fig. 8.25A,B.

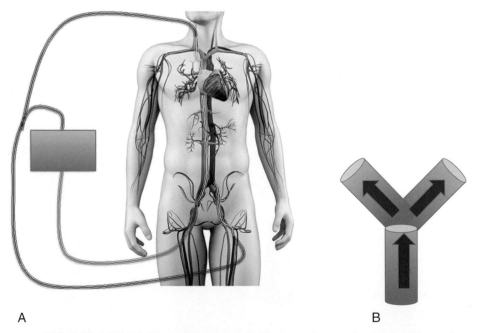

FIG. 8.25 VAV hybrid configuration with Y connection on the return side (Modified from SciePro/Shutterstock.com.)

This tends to be a more common configuration because there is a physiologic rationale for providing antegrade oxygenated blood in peripherally placed VA ECMO, where there may be the possibility of deoxygenated, competing flow that is being ejected by the heart. We will dive into this physiology in much more detail when we further explore retrograde physiology in Chapter 14.

A FINAL WORD

We covered a lot of configurations in this chapter. Some you may commonly come across, while some can be rarely employed based on the physiologic result that is trying to be achieved. In either case, this emphasizes the importance of thoughtful consideration behind cannula selection and configuration. The team managing a patient on ECMO should have a prediction of what physiology they are likely to encounter and proceed accordingly with the appropriately sized cannulas and configuration.

Keep in mind, there is something to be said for simplicity and consistency. If you are able to achieve your anticipated physiologic endpoints, choosing cannula sizes and configurations that you are comfortable with understanding and managing can be prudent.

SUGGESTED READING

Aggarwal, V., Einhorn, B. N., & Cohen, H. A. (2016). Current status of percutaneous right ventricular assist devices: first-in-man use of a novel dual lumen cannula. *Catheterization and Cardiovascular Interventions*, 88(3), 390–396.

Brasseur, A., Scolletta, S., Lorusso, R., & Taccone, F. S. (2018). Hybrid extracorporeal membrane oxygenation. *Journal of Thoracic Disease*, 10(Suppl 5), S707.

Burrell, A. J. C., Ihle, J. F., Pellegrino, V. A., Sheldrake, J., & Nixon, P. T. (2018). Cannulation technique: femoro-femoral. *Journal of Thoracic Disease*, 10(Suppl 5), S616.

Javidfar, J., Brodie, D., Wang, D., Ibrahimiye, A. N., Yang, J., & Zwischenberger, J. B., et al. (2011). Use of bicaval dual-lumen catheter for adult venovenous extracorporeal membrane oxygenation. *The Annals of Thoracic Surgery*, 91(6), 1763–1769.

Juo, Y. Y., Skancke, M., Sanaiha, Y., Mantha, A., Jimenez, J. C., & Benharash, P., et al. (2017). Efficacy of distal perfusion cannulae in preventing limb ischemia during extracorporeal membrane oxygenation: a systematic review and meta-analysis. *Artificial Organs*, 41(11), E263–E273.

Palmér, O., Palmér, K., Hultman, J., & Broman, M. (2016). Cannula design and recirculation during venovenous extracorporeal membrane oxygenation. *ASAIO Journal*, 62(6), 737.

9

Components, Sensors, and Circuit Access

Now that we have a little more foundation, let's return to our circuit, and dive a little deeper into the circuit components that you may come across and how you may interact with them (Fig. 9.1).

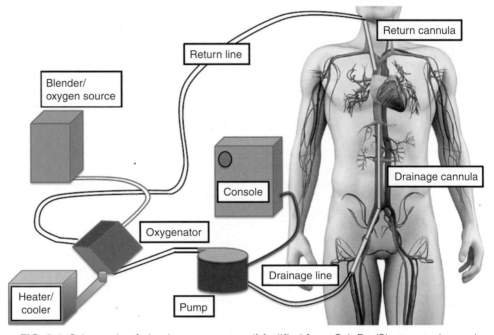

FIG. 9.1 Schematic of circuit components. (Modified from SciePro/Shutterstock.com.)

TUBING

The tubing is the conduit by which the blood flows through to the various components, namely the pump and oxygenator. Tubing is made of a flexible, clear, plastic that allows visualization of the color of blood as well as any areas of potential turbulence or clot.

Circuits can be built to different specifications, but the standard for adults usually includes tubing with a diameter of 3/8″. This width is wide enough to minimize resistance to flow while not requiring an excessive amount of extracorporeal blood. Some pediatric circuits and low-flow extracorporeal membrane oxygenation (ECMO) circuits may take advantage of smaller tubing such as 1/4″, which allows for less circulating blood but may have some impedance of flow.

The length of the tubing can vary – usually the standard is around 15 feet. You may encounter circuits with longer or shorter tubing. The main advantage of longer tubing is less constraint of having to be close to the circuit, but this should be compared to the disadvantages to include more length to monitor, more possibilities for occlusion, and higher priming volume.

3/8" tubing carries about 20 mL per foot, meaning that a circuit with 15 feet of tubing has a priming volume of 300 mL plus the priming volume of the oxygenator (usually around 250–300 mL). The priming volume is important for several reasons:

1. It represents the dilutional volume when going on ECMO.
2. It represents the amount of blood lost when a circuit is lost or changed.
3. It represents the increase in volume of distribution to be considered for pharmacokinetics and effect of medications.

PUMP

We were introduced to the blood pump in Chapter 6, now let's go a little deeper into what it involves. Blood pumps were traditionally roller pumps, which milked the blood forward; however, these have been largely replaced by centrifugal pumps in adults.

Although there are many different models of centrifugal pump, the central mechanism is a cone or a fin that spins around in a centrifugal manner. This pump head is connected to a motor that drives this rotation (Fig. 9.2).

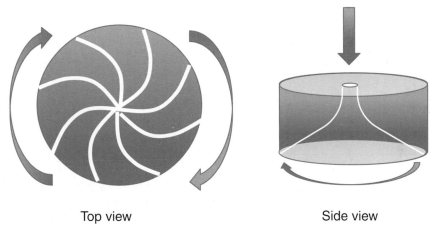

Top view   Side view

FIG. 9.2 Centrifugal pump

The result is a creation of a vortex of blood that is pulled in through the top and pushed out through the bottom as illustrated in Fig. 9.3.

This pull/push mechanism by which blood enters/exits the pump is an essential part to understanding the flow dynamics related to ECMO, so let's reflect on it.

> Because of the rotational mechanism of the centrifugal pump, any blood going **into** the pump will be under **negative** pressure, while any blood **leaving** the pump will be under **positive** pressure.

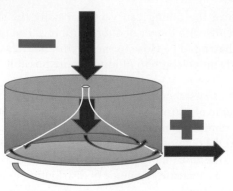

FIG. 9.3 Blood flow through centrifugal pump with negative pressure at the inlet and positive pressure at the outlet

We will go into how this affects the flow of blood in much greater detail in Chapter 10, when we cover flow dynamics. For now, we can start to appreciate how this phenomenon will affect the flow of blood and how we can approach the circuit.

Essence of Centrifugal Pump: Preload Dependence and Afterload Sensitivity

Because the centrifugal pump generates a negative pressure on the inlet and positive pressure on the outlet, you have preload dependence and afterload sensitivity. This means that the availability of blood going to the pump (preload) is requisite for the pump to work, while impedance of flow (afterload) will result in a decrease in the forward flow of blood.

To better visualize afterload sensitivity, think of a boat that is parked in front of a dock. The propeller can spin as fast as you would like; however, if there is a barrier in front of the boat (the dock in this case), there will be no forward movement. The same is true with the centrifugal pump. If you kink or clamp the outflow line, the pump will keep spinning at the same number of revolutions per minute (RPMs), but the flow will drop off.

This represents a major differentiator from roller pumps, where an occlusion downstream from the pump will only cause pressures to increase, as the forward flow of blood will be relatively fixed.

There are two major implications of this afterload sensitivity, the first being that flow will be impacted by the pressure that exists downstream of the pump. This could be anything that impedes flow such as a clot in the oxygenator, a kink in the return line, a bend in the return cannula, or an elevation in the systemic blood pressure if on VA ECMO. The remedy for this would be to fix any of these impediments to flow or to increase the RPMs in an attempt to overcome this afterload and optimize flow (Fig. 9.4).

The second implication of the afterload sensitivity of the centrifugal pump is that the pump can be subjected to **retrograde flow** at lower RPMs while on VA ECMO. Why is this? Let's consider an example to illustrate.

Say you are decreasing the RPMs down to lower the blood flow on a patient who is slowly recovering with improving blood pressure. As you continue to decrease the RPMs, eventually, the afterload of the patient's mean arterial pressure (MAP) drops the flow to 0. At this point, there exists a higher pressure on the return side of the pump than on the drainage side (as the MAP is higher than the venous pressure), and you will get retrograde flow from the arterial system to the venous system, as illustrated in Fig. 9.5.

The clinical implication of this is that if your RPMs drop below a critical threshold, you can induce a left to right shunt, which can cause a rapid decompensation.

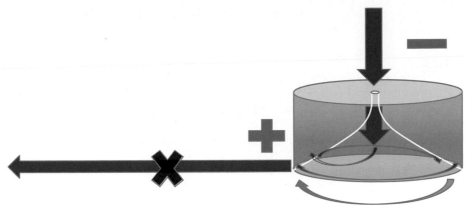

FIG. 9.4 Afterload sensitivity: anything that increases pressure downstream from the pump can impact overall flow

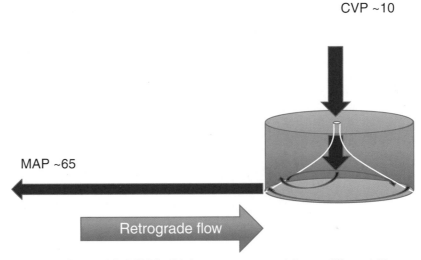

FIG. 9.5 Retrograde flow on VA ECMO with lower pump speed due to differential between arterial and venous pressures. *CVP*, Central venous pressure; *MAP*, mean arterial pressure.

MECHANICAL BACKUP

If our discussion of the pump does anything, it should highlight how bad things can get if the circuit stops flowing. Let's review why:

1. Drop in the flow of oxygenated blood in a patient who may be dependent on the oxygenated blood to maintain delivery of oxygen
2. Lack of blood flow in a patient who may be dependent on that flow to maintain cardiac output
3. Retrograde flow with worsening of the right to left shunt and infusion of venous blood into arterial circulation (on VA ECMO)
4. Stagnation of blood with thrombus formation

   Taken together, these may lead to cardiac arrest and rapid deterioration.

   Having a strategy to mitigate pump failure is paramount. Ensure there is a backup for power failure, whether it is a hand crank or a backup console next to the pump at all times. This includes during procedures, transport to anywhere in the hospital, physical therapy, etc. That is one thing about emergencies – they always seem to happen when we are least prepared!

CONSOLE

We discovered during our initial introduction to the console that in its most basic form, it is a mechanism for manipulating RPMs to the pump via connection with the electric motor and a display of flow and RPMs. The mechanism for increasing/decreasing RPMs can be a push button or a dial, with the convention being clockwise rotation to increase RPMs and counterclockwise rotation to decrease RPMs.

You are probably arriving to the conclusion that there are many determinants of blood flow (we will continue to develop these concepts in Chapter 10). Thus, RPMs are set by the console and transmitted to the motor/pump. The flow that is obtained by these RPMs has to be measured directly.

SENSORS: MEASURING ECMO SUPPORT

The way that blood flow is measured during ECMO support is by direct measurement through sensor probes. This is one advantage of having a support device with blood that is circulated outside the body – by contrast, ventricular support devices determine flow by a calculated algorithm as there is nothing to measure directly.

Flow sensors are circumferential sensors that surround the tubing and are connected to the console. They are placed on the return tubing and must be oriented in the same direction as the blood is flowing. If the sensor probe is on backwards, the console will read a negative flow rate (Fig. 9.6).

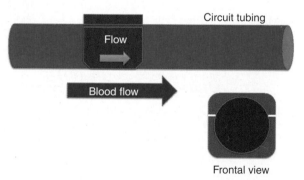

FIG. 9.6 Flow sensor probe

They function by sending sonographic signals to each pole, which are disrupted in proportion to the flow of blood. The faster the flow of blood the greater the reduction of waves moving against that flow and the greater the augmentation of waves moving with the flow of blood as illustrated in Fig. 9.7. The degree of augmentation/reduction of these waves is used to calculate a flow of blood.

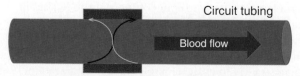

FIG. 9.7 Mechanism of flow sensor

Sensors can also be used to measure hemoglobin or the presence of air in the circuit. Air is measured through the disruption of sonographic waves, which normally pass from one side of the sensor to the other uninterrupted (Fig. 9.8).

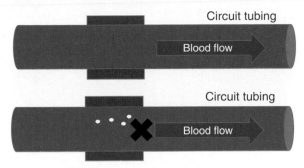

FIG 9.8 Mechanism of air sensor

The effect of this depends on how the console is set, either to alarm or for intervention. As the intervention usually involves stopping the pump, the decision on whether or not interventions should be set involves an evaluation of the risks of air versus the risks of pump stoppage. Regardless, consistency should predominate.

CIRCUIT ACCESS POINTS

At its most basic form, everything we have covered to this point makes for a complete circuit. We have covered all of the essential components. For some programs, this is extent of the circuit. However, most circuits have access points where the circuit can be accessed, which allows for blood draws, medication administration, continuous renal replacement therapy (CRRT) connections, and pressure monitoring. These come in the form of pigtail connections as seen in Fig. 9.9.

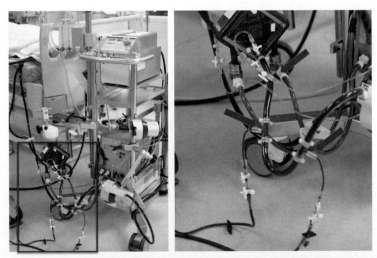

FIG 9.9 Circuit access points. (From PIJITRA PHOMKHAM/Shutterstock.com.)

Let's simplify our circuit illustration, as there really are only a few spots in the circuit where there can be access points: pre-pump, post-pump/pre-oxygenator, and post-oxygenator as illustrated in Fig. 9.10.

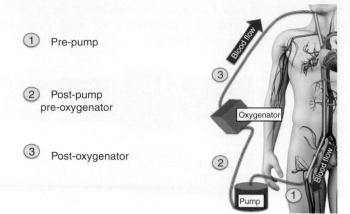

1. Pre-pump

2. Post-pump
   pre-oxygenator

3. Post-oxygenator

FIG. 9.10 Potential circuit access points. (Modified from SciePro/Shutterstock.com.)

Let's review each individually:

1. **Pre-pump**. Beware of this hookup! Remember, this is under negative pressure, so any time you access it, it air can be entrained. Entrained air can deprime your oxygenator, air lock (and stop) your pump, or embolize to the patient. The negative pressure can allow for quick administration of fluid blood but may be a risky proposition.

2. **Post-pump/pre-oxygenator**. This is your safety zone (or at least your *safer* zone). It is positive pressure, but you have an oxygenator between your access and the patient, which could potentially "catch" any air/clot that gets pushed through the access.

3. **Post-oxygenator**. This access point is also under positive pressure but is a little more risky, since there is no oxygenator between any clot or air that gets administered to the circuit.

Some ECMO programs have multiple points of access to the circuit while some have none. Just remember that the more you access the circuit, the greater the risk for bleeding, alarms, embolization, or potentially air entrainment. Ultimately, it becomes a matter of risk/benefit – what gives enough capabilities but limits the risk of an adverse event.

Let's now go over several indications for accessing the circuit.

Access Point Indication #1: Medication/Blood/Fluid Administration

If you were going to choose one position to administer to the circuit, it would be post-pump/pre-oxygenator (position 2 in Fig. 9.11). This site allows for positive pressure and allows the oxygenator to stand in the way of any air or clot that happens to be entrained. Anticoagulation can also be administered here, which theoretically could help to minimize clot formation on the oxygenator.

Access Point Indication #2: Blood Gas Draws

If you are drawing blood gases for a patient on ECMO, there are three positions from which you will draw: pre-oxygenator, post-oxygenator, and from the patient (blue arrows in Fig. 9.12). We will discuss the rationale more in Chapter 11 as well as some techniques for interpreting these gases. For now, suffice it to say that checking circuit gases both pre-oxygenator and post-oxygenator allows us to diagnose issues and evaluate the circuit.

Access Point Indication #3: Pressure Monitoring

Pressure monitoring can give important data on how to manage the circuit. Pressures can be transduced in any of our positions, and can help to diagnose and manage issues related to the pump. Remember that position 1 is negative pressure, so usually it is only transduced if it is an integrated sensor that minimizes the risk for access to the negative side of the circuit.

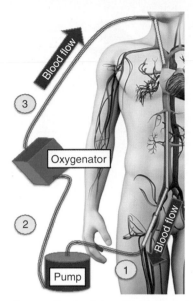

FIG. 9.11 Circuit access for medication/blood/fluid administration. (Modified from SciePro/Shutterstock.com.)

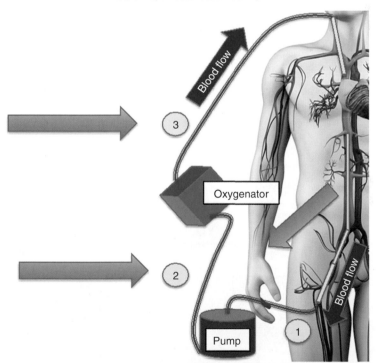

FIG. 9.12 Sites to draw blood gas samples on ECMO: patient arterial line, post oxygenator, and pre oxygenator. (Modified from SciePro/Shutterstock.com.)

The anticipated pressures are as illustrated in Fig. 9.13.

Point 1 is the lowest pressure in the system. Remember that the centrifugal pump generates the flow for the entire system, so you should anticipate the most negative pressure measured to be right before the pump and the highest pressure generated to be right after the pump. Pressure

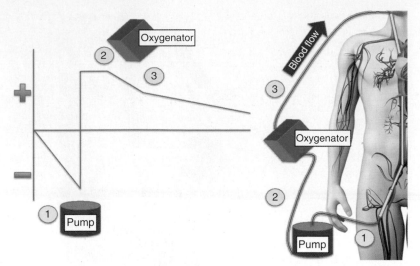

FIG. 9.13 Schematic of circuit pressures relative to ECMO pump and oxygenator. (Modified from SciePro/Shutterstock.com.)

should gradually decrease the further you get from the pump, with a distinct drop-off between point 2 and point 3, which represents the pressure differential across the oxygenator. We will go into the interpretation of these pressure differentials more in the next two chapters.

Access Point Indication #4: CRRT Connection

CRRT and dialysis can be connected directly to the ECMO circuit, obviating the need for a separate catheter. Connecting CRRT can be another point that differs between ECMO programs – some prefer to minimize access to the circuit and always place a separate catheter, some find it a convenient way to initiate renal replacement (Fig. 9.14).

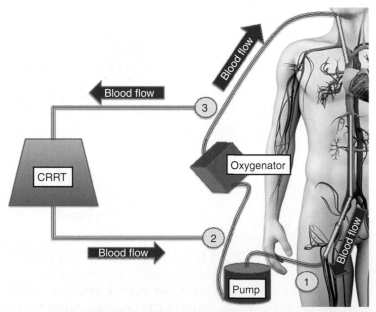

FIG. 9.14 Example connection for continuous renal replacement therapy. (Modified from SciePro/Shutterstock.com.). *CRRT,* Continuous renal replacement therapy.

Some dialysis machines may work better with different connections based on the pressure differential; however, all else being equal, connecting from post-oxygenator to pre-oxygenator allows an additional element of safety by putting the oxygenator between blood that is returning and the patient, allowing for a potential barrier for any air/thrombus that gets returned by the dialysis circuit.

THE CIRCUIT CHECK: THE MOST IMPORTANT PART OF YOUR DAY

Now that we have gone in depth for all of the components of the ECMO circuit, let's introduce one of the most fundamental practices in the management of any patient on ECMO – the circuit check.

The circuit check involves a tip-to-tip inspection of the entire circuit with attention to all of its components.

A Word of Advice on the Circuit Check

Often, when team members perform circuit checks, they do a quick runthrough of the circuit, making some cursory glances at some components. This approach is sure to miss something. Consider treating the circuit check like a pilot treats her preflight checklist. She may have done it thousands of times but uses a checklist to ensure every part of every component of the list is accounted for. The following is a proposed checklist for how to run a circuit check. Remember, practice doesn't make perfect – perfect practice makes perfect!

Be diligent, be purposeful, be consistent.

Checklist for Circuit Check

☐ Cart–at least 6 clamps, full O_2 tank, supplies for emergency circuit change, hand crank/backup console

☐ Console–plugged into appropriate electrical receptacle, alarms activated, interventions set as appropriate

☐ Oxygen blender–connected to O_2 tank or wall O_2/medical air

☐ Heater/cooler–plugged into appropriate electrical receptacle, water level filled, hoses/connectors free of kinks and leaks

☐ Drain cannula–dressing clean/dry, suture present and intact, connector intact

☐ Drain line–free of clots/fibrin build up/defects

☐ Drain line connectors–secure, free of leaks, inspected for fibrin buildup

☐ Pump–inflow and outflow free from obstruction/fibrin buildup

☐ Pre oxygenator–systematically check for clots/fibrin buildup

☐ Pre oxygenator pigtails–patent, stopcocks oriented in correct position, clamps intact

☐ Oxygenator–exhaust free from obstruction, green O_2 tubing connected to appropriate gas source, water lines connected and free of leaks

☐ Post oxygenator–systematically check for clots and fibrin build up

☐ Post oxygenator pigtails–patent, stopcocks oriented in correct position, clamps intact

☐ Flow probe/bubble detector–connected, activated as appropriate, free of line defects

☐ SvO_2 probe–connected, free of line defects

☐ Return line–free of clots/fibrin buildup/defects

☐ Return line connectors–secure, free of leaks, inspected for fibrin buildup

☐ Return cannula–dressing clean/dry, suture present and intact, connector intact

SUGGESTED READING

de Tymowski, C., Augustin, P., Houissa, H., Allou, N., Montravers, P., & Delzongle, A., et al. (2017). CRRT connected to ECMO: managing high pressures. *ASAIO Journal*, *63*(1), 48–52.

Lawson, D. S., Ing, R., Cheifetz, I. M., Walczak, R., Craig, D., & Schulman, S., et al. (2005). Hemolytic characteristics of three commercially available centrifugal blood pumps. *Pediatric Critical Care Medicine*, *6*(5), 573–577.

Pedersen, T. H., Videm, V., Svennevig, J. L., Karlsen, H., Ostbakk, R. W., & Jensen, O., et al. (1997). Extracorporeal membrane oxygenation using a centrifugal pump and a servo regulator to prevent negative inlet pressure. *The Annals of Thoracic Surgery*, *63*(5), 1333–1339.

Westrope, C., Harvey, C., Robinson, S., Speggiorin, S., Faulkner, G., & Peek, G. J., et al. (2013). Pump controlled retrograde trial off from VA-ECMO. *ASAIO Journal*, *59*(5), 517–519.

PART III

ECMO Physiology

10

Blood Flow Dynamics

We are now going to continue our journey by exploring the physiology of extracorporeal membrane oxygenation (ECMO) support. You may find the chapters to follow to be the cornerstone of the understanding of ECMO. It is a common adage to hear the following:

"ECMO is easy to initiate, the challenge is in the management."

I fully agree with this sentiment, but the challenge in management is rarely what we think. The stalwarts of good critical care support remain consistent – medications, antibiotics, nutrition, and rehabilitation. However, the true challenge in managing patients on ECMO involves developing an appreciation, understanding, and familiarity with the physiology of extracorporeal support – the following chapters will be aimed to equip you with the tools needed to do just that.

Let's start by developing our understanding of the limits of blood flow and the ECMO circuit.

WHY IS BLOOD FLOW SO ESSENTIAL IN ECMO SUPPORT?

You will recall that there are two primary parameters that can be manipulated in ECMO support: **sweep gas flow**, which contributes to ventilation/CO_2 removal, and **blood flow**, which primarily contributes to oxygenation.

Why is this the case? Shouldn't support just be support? Shouldn't a higher oxygenated gas flow just increase oxygenation?

To answer this, we will have to return to our first chapter on the physiology of oxygen delivery.

Remember when it really comes to oxygen *delivery*, the ultimate determinant is hemoglobin, because hemoglobin is just so much better at delivering oxygen due to its ability to bind oxygen with increasing affinity in the heart lungs as well as the ability to change forms to and dump oxygen in the periphery (Fig. 10.1).

We covered in great detail what this means for the body in terms of delivering oxygen – that the better we can leverage the efficiency of hemoglobin, through optimizing saturation/hemoglobin/cardiac output, the better we can deliver oxygen.

Now let's apply this concept in the context of the ECMO circuit. You will recall for delivery of oxygen in the body we have the following equation:

$$DO_2 = 1.34 \times SaO_2 \times Hb \times CO + PaO_2 \times 0.003$$

which can be simplified to the following relationship:

$$DO_2 \rightarrow SaO_2 \times Hb \times CO$$

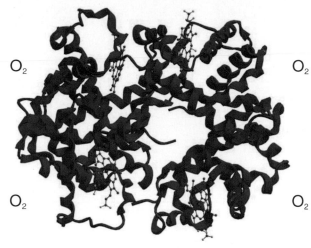

FIG. 10.1 Hemoglobin as a means of delivering oxygen. (From Raimundo79/Shutterstock.com.)

For the delivery of oxygen by the ECMO circuit, the determinants become oxygen saturation, hemoglobin, and instead of cardiac output, the blood flow through the ECMO circuit (Fig. 10.2).

Oxygenator DO_2 ⇨ Blood flow × Hb × SO_2

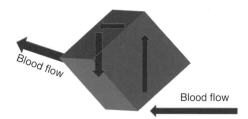

FIG. 10.2 Oxygen delivery capability of the oxygenator

WHAT ABOUT FiO₂?

Doesn't increasing FiO_2 improve the delivery of oxygen to the ECMO circuit much the same way that increasing FiO_2 administered to the lungs can increase oxygen delivery? Yes and no. The FiO_2 dial on the blender alters the amount of oxygen running through the oxygenator and drives the gradient at the membrane level, but ultimately, it does not matter how much oxygen diffuses across (otherwise known as your PaO_2); what ultimately matters to the delivery of oxygen is the saturation of hemoglobin by that oxygen.

At a certain point, it does not matter how high the PaO_2 of the blood coming out of the oxygenator is, there is a maximum saturation after which hemoglobin does not get much more saturated and the hemoglobin saturation curve flattens out (Fig. 10.3).

The oxygenator is very good at saturating blood, and there is rarely a problem with maintaining adequate saturation of blood coming out of the oxygenator. Rather at this point, we can start to appreciate that the determinants of oxygen delivery of the oxygenator are saturation of the

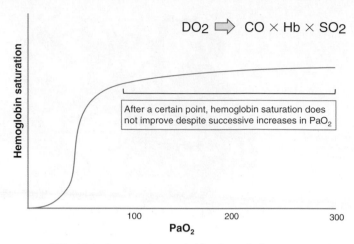

FIG. 10.3 Oxygen hemoglobin dissociation curve

blood coming out of the oxygenator (largely expected to be 100%), hemoglobin concentration, and, ultimately, the blood flow coming out of the oxygenator to the extent that we are able to provide this flow.

So more blood flow, better oxygen delivery – sounds easy enough. If you need more oxygen delivery, you provide more blood flow, right? As we will see, the ability to provide flow has been limited both by the pump/circuit and by the body.

WHAT ARE THE DETERMINANTS OF BLOOD FLOW ON ECMO SUPPORT?

Said another way, what limits our ECMO blood flow? We will discuss how we can titrate ECMO blood flow in Chapter 17, but for now, let's focus only on the limits to blood flow. As we will discover, there are a host of limits to blood flow ranging from patient factors to factors associated with the circuit.

LIMITS OF THE MEMBRANE OXYGENATOR

Seems like with all of this technology and capability, the membrane oxygenator will be much better at oxygenation than our lungs, right? Actually, the oxygenator doesn't even come close to the potential capability of the lungs. Ultimately, it all comes down to the blood/gas interface. With the lungs, that interface comes in the form of the blood/alveolar interface. That means that the surface area of the 600 million alveoli in the lungs comes out to around 150 m^2, roughly the size of a tennis court. Compare this to the 4 m^2 surface area of the plastic fibers of most oxygenators, barely half of one of the service boxes. Additionally this interface is approximately 10–20 times thicker for the oxygenator than for the lungs, further hindering the diffusion of oxygen (Fig. 10.4).

Additionally, blood does not flow smoothly through the oxygenator, rather, it experiences a decrease in laminar flow both on the macro and micro levels as illustrated in Fig. 10.5.

As seen on the left, there will be areas throughout the oxygenator, such as right angles, corners, and any place where the flow of blood changes direction, where the flow of blood will slow down, giving rise to turbulence and ultimately decreasing the efficiency of the blood flow. The right illustrates how this can happen at the level of the plastic fibers, with blood changing direction to flow past the individual fibers.

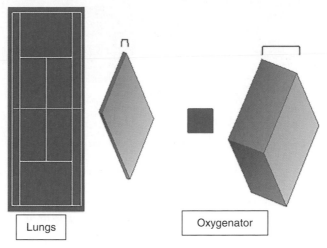

FIG. 10.4 Oxygenation capability of native lungs versus membrane oxygenator

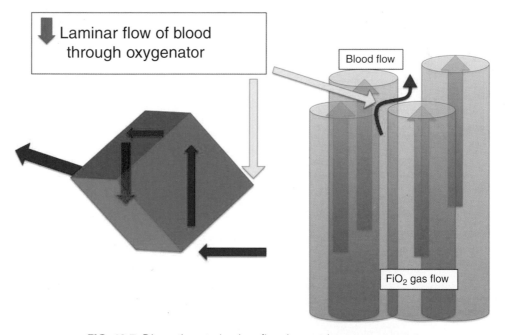

FIG. 10.5 Disruptions to laminar flow in membrane oxygenator

EFFECT OF MEMBRANE LIMITS: THE RATED FLOW OF THE MEMBRANE

With these inefficiencies and limits, we should be able to imagine how these add up to a maximum amount of flow that the membrane can tolerate, past which there would be no further increase in the content of blood (CaO_2) provided by the oxygenator (where $CaO_2 = 1.34 \times SaO_2 \times Hb + PaO_2 \times 0.003$) (Fig. 10.6).

Any further increase in blood flow past this maximum flow would just represent shunt, much in the same way that shunted blood in the lungs represents blood that shunts across without participating in gas exchange.

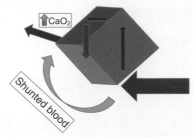

FIG. 10.6 Higher blood flow increases the proportion of shunted blood across the oxygenator

Let's now try to conceptualize what this looks like when it comes to how blood flows through an oxygenator. Imagine that you have an oxygenator with blood flowing through it with no limit on the amount of blood that can flow. If we were to plot the relationship between this blood flow and the oxygen content of the blood leaving the oxygenator, we would conceptualize something like what is shown in Fig. 10.7.

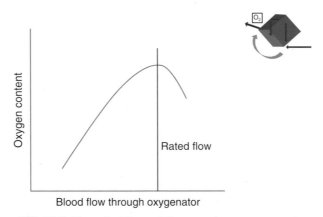

FIG. 10.7 The rated flow of the membrane oxygenator

In this graph, we see that at the beginning, as blood flow increases, the oxygen content would increase precipitously at first, then taper off as we approach the red line, due to shunting. However, as we continue to increase the blood flow, there reaches a critical point (red line), where the CaO_2 of blood leaving the oxygenator actually *decreases*, as the amount of shunted blood exceeds the non-shunted blood going through the oxygenator.

This point, where blood flow corresponds with the maximum content of oxygen that can be delivered, is referred to as the **rated flow** of the membrane.

Although every oxygenator that is being used clinically will perform differently depending on the age of the oxygenator, the level of anticoagulation, or the coagulation status of the blood, the rated flow, is a manufacturer-specified attribute, that is standard to all membrane oxygenators.

Since the rated flow represents the blood flow corresponding with the maximum CaO_2, it will usually be listed in the context of a standard hemoglobin and saturation change, with the convention that flow can raise the saturation of preoxygenator blood from 75% to 95% at a hemoglobin concentration of 12 g/dL.

BLOOD FLOW LIMITS OF THE CIRCUIT

So far, we have been discussing the limits of the membrane oxygenator with the assumption that there are no limits to blood flow in and out of the oxygenator. Now, let's consider the determinants of this blood flow and how these determinants drive and limit blood flow.

To further understand the dynamics of flow through a closed system, let's imagine two balloons filled with fluid, with Balloon 1 being completely filled up and Balloon 2 being empty, such that the pressure in Balloon 1 (P1) is much greater than the pressure in Balloon 2 (P2).

Now, let's connect these two balloons with some tubing. As you would imagine, there would be a flow of fluid in the direction of P1 to P2. What would determine the rate of flow? First, the pressure differential between the two balloons (P1 – P2) would play a large role. The more pressure the contents of Balloon 1 are under, the greater the flow of fluid (Fig. 10.8).

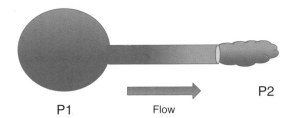

FIG. 10.8 Determinants of flow through a closed system

Past this point, the flow will be determined by the characteristics of the fluid and the tube connecting the two balloons. The thicker the fluid, the less flow you would anticipate. Additionally, the longer the tubing that connects the two balloons, the less flow, while the wider the tubing, the higher the flow.

This relationship of flow through a closed system is exactly what is happening in our ECMO circuit. Let's now apply these concepts to the circuit, drawing some conclusions that will be relevant to our clinical understanding and decision-making.

The standard equation for accounting for these variables when it comes to flow through a closed system is as follows:

$$\text{Flow} = \frac{\pi \times \Delta P \times r^4}{8 \times \text{viscosity} \times \text{length}}$$

Let's now put these variables into the context of the ECMO circuit. When we consider blood flow through an ECMO circuit, we have:

> **ΔP:** pressure differential driven by the centrifugal pump and across circuit
> **r:** width of cannulas and tubing (lesser extent)
> **length:** length of tubing and cannulas (lesser extent)
> **viscosity:** hematocrit and hemoconcentration

PRESSURE DIFFERENTIAL: ROLE OF CENTRIFUGAL PUMP

Remember in the example of our balloons, the greater the pressure differential, the greater the flow is. This is the essence behind the centrifugal pump that we introduced in Chapter 9.

To remind ourselves, the centrifugal pump consists of cones/fins that spin, creating a vortex, that *pulls* blood in through negative pressure and *pushes* the blood out through positive pressure (Fig. 10.9).

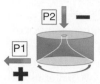

FIG. 10.9 The pressure differential generated by the centrifugal pump

The faster the pump spins, greater is the negative pressure generated (P2), and greater is the positive pressure generated (P1). Therefore, as the pump speed increases with higher revolutions per minute (RPMs), ΔP (P1 – P2) will also increase with a consequent increase in flow.

This increase in flow however, is limited by the **preload dependence** and **afterload sensitivity** of the centrifugal pump. Let's explore these concepts, which are fundamental to the centrifugal pump.

Effect of Preload Dependence on Pump Flow

Preload dependence is a distinct limit of the centrifugal pump. Just like the effect of preload on the cardiac myocytes introduced in Chapter 2, preload represents the filling pressure of the drainage system. This preload translates into the availability of blood for drainage necessary for the flow of blood through the pump.

This dependence on preload is even more profound for the centrifugal pump than for the heart due to the nature of the negative pressure generated by the pump. Even a modest drop in the pressure of blood in the venous drainage system (represented by central venous pressure [CVP]) can cause the pump flows to drop precipitously. Clinically, this means that often a drop in ECMO flows can precede a drop in mean arterial pressure (MAP) in the presence of hypovolemia.

There are two primary factors that determine the preload/filling pressures of the pump; the drainage cannula and the venous system from which the pump is draining blood.

Drainage Cannula

The drainage cannula can limit blood that can be pulled into the pump. The bigger the drainage cannula, the better the potential flow of blood. This is why the selection of the type/size/position of the drainage cannula is so important to the flow of blood and should always be considered when selecting cannulas at the beginning of an ECMO run. As you may recall from our discussion of cannula types, the typical drainage cannula is a multistage cannula, with multiple drainage holes throughout the length of the cannula that allow for increased flow relative to the negative pressure generated (Fig. 10.10).

Pressure of the Venous System

The number of drainage holes and size/position of the drainage cannula determine the negative pressure required to drain a specific volume of blood. This pressure is then exerted on the pressure of the venous system that the cannula is positioned in. If there is sufficient venous pressure, then the blood will be drained easily, facilitating blood flow into the pump.

However, if there is insufficient venous pressure (due to hypovolemia, a malpositioned cannula outside of the intrahepatic inferior vena cava (IVC), or increased abdominal pressures due to coughing as examples), then the negative pressure generated from the pump will be exerted onto

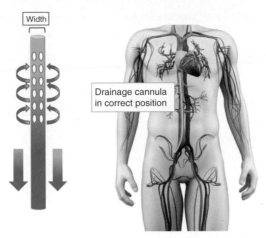

FIG. 10.10 Effect of drainage cannula size and position on pump filling pressures. (Modified from SciePro/Shutterstock.com.)

the vessel wall, causing it to suck down (position A to position B below), before returning to normal (position C) as flows drop (Fig. 10.11A–C).

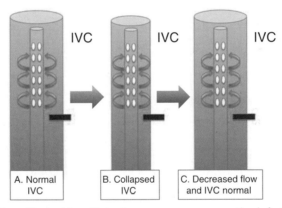

FIG. 10.11 The effect of insufficient venous pressure on the inferior vena cava
IVC, Inferior vena cava

The insufficient venous pressure causes a rapid drop in flow due to the unavailability of preload, which in turn decreases the negative pressure and releases the pressure exerted on the vessel wall. This process can repeat itself, causing the lines to jump and flows to fluctuate up and down, which is commonly referred to as "chatter."

The take home point is that preload is essential for the centrifugal pump to work. Without adequate filling pressures, the pump cannot generate a pressure differential, and flows will drop precipitously.

Effect of Afterload Sensitivity on Pump Flow

Let's now turn our attention to the positive pressure side of the pump. You will recall from our discussion of the pump in Chapter 9, we introduced the concept of afterload sensitivity, which stated that increased pressure downstream of the pump introduces afterload that the pump must push against.

As illustrated in Fig. 10.12, afterload decreases the gradient between P1 and P2.

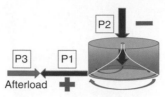

FIG. 10.12 The effect of afterload to the centrifugal pump on blood flow

The ultimate effect of this is a drop in ΔP, which will lead to an overall reduction in flow, as follows:

$$\Delta P = (P1 - P3) - P2$$

What Represents Afterload to the ECMO Pump?

Anything that increases pressure on the positive side of the pump can influence afterload. This includes the oxygenator, the return line, any additional source of increased resistance in this system (connectors/clots kinks/occlusions), and, ultimately, the pressure of the vascular system to which the blood is being returned.

If you are on VV ECMO, you are returning blood to the venous system and the afterload contribution of that system is the pressure of the venous system (~CVP). Contrast this to VA ECMO, where the afterload contribution of the vascular system is the pressure of the arterial system (~MAP), which you can anticipate to be much higher. Therefore, afterload sensitivity will be a bigger consideration for VA ECMO.

What Are the Clinical Implications of Afterload Sensitivity?

The pressure differential generated by the centrifugal pump always has to overcome this afterload, otherwise, retrograde flow will ensue. How can you mitigate this clinically when managing the patient, especially on VA ECMO?

1. When initiating ECMO, start with a fixed number of RPMs (usually around 1500) so that forward flow is maintained.
2. When weaning blood flows, maintain some RPMs so that you are evaluating lower flows, without experiencing retrograde flow.
3. If the pump stops flowing, clamp the circuit so that you will not have retrograde flow.
   We will explore these more in the management section.

THE EFFECT OF RESISTANCE AND THE LIMITATION OF FLOW

We should now have a good sense of the effect of pressure differential (ΔP) on flow. Let's now turn towards the resistance of the system, and the effect that it has on overall flow. Resistance represents the other variables we identified in our system: radius, viscosity, and length as represented in our equation:

$$\text{Flow} = \frac{\pi \Delta P r^4}{8 \times \text{viscosity} \times \text{length}}$$

We will go over each of these and how they manifest in the ECMO circuit.

Radius and Limitations to Flow

Of the three variables, the radius of the system has the most significant effect on flow. That is why it is represented as r^4, signifying that any increase in the radius increases the flow by a factor to the fourth power. As an example, doubling the radius translates to a 16-fold increase in flow. Let's consider the effect of radius on flow as it relates to cannula size.

As an example, if you are trying to select between a 10-French cannula and a 25-French drainage cannula, you may be tempted to select the 19-French cannula, maybe to lessen the risk of venous obstruction, lower extremity compartment syndrome, or need for further dilation. You may rationalize that this only translates into a 2-mm change in diameter. However, this move actually translates into a three fold reduction in overall flow that the drainage cannula can accommodate! This highlights the importance of factoring in the role of radius of your circuit into the anticipated flow.

Length and Limitations to Flow

In a similar fashion, the longer the length of your system, the more resistance there is to flow. Let's return to our system connecting the two balloons. First imagine the flow between the balloons if the tubing connecting them was a foot. Now, imagine it is a mile long – you can envision the flow of fluid being significantly reduced, right (Fig. 10.13)?

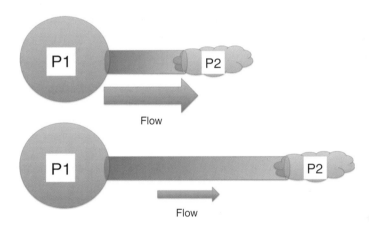

FIG. 10.13 The effect of length on flow

This becomes very relevant for the ECMO circuit. When building your circuit, you may come up with all kinds of reasons to build in more length – allow for greater mobility, facilitate transport, allow the patient to be pushed through the CT scanner, etc. Many of these are clinically essential. However, keep in mind the effect of length on overall flow.

Viscosity and Limitations to Flow

The primary determinant of viscosity is hematocrit, which can reflect red blood cells as well as hemoconcentration. For the most part, hematocrit/viscosity has a minimal effect on flow, as the level of hematocrit needed to have an appreciable effect on viscosity and ultimately flow becomes clinically untenable. If we were to plot the relationship of hematocrit to viscosity, we would have something similar to (Fig. 10.14), with a minimal effect on viscosity at levels seen in most patients, and an escalation in viscosity at levels of hemoglobin rarely seen in the critically ill patient population.

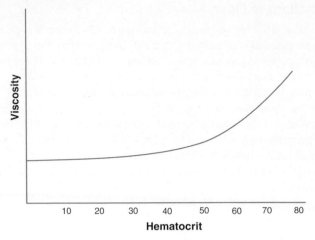

FIG. 10.14 The effect of hematocrit on viscosity

RPM Limits to Flow

We have now covered limits to flow as they relate to a theoretical closed system, but there are additional limits that are worth considering. The first is the limit of RPMs themselves. As a centrifugal pump spins at higher and higher speeds, you may not have any limitations to flow in terms of the rated flow of the membrane, preload dependence/afterload sensitivity of the pump, or resistance of the circuit.

However, at these high speeds, you may have a limitation due to the damaging effects of high RPMs on the blood that is being circulated through the pump. Specifically, high pump speeds can cause trauma to the red blood cells, manifesting as hemolysis. Besides the potential loss of blood cells, this hemolysis can cause a variety of adverse effects including renal toxicity, reduced immune function, potential for thrombosis, and alterations in hemodynamics.

Potential effects to monitor for hemolysis due to high pump speeds include jaundice, elevated plasma-free hemoglobin, elevated lactate dehydrogenase, elevated bilirubin, and dark urine. The presence of any of these may be a sign that RPMs are limiting or at the very least, should be limiting flow.

Effect of Recirculation Limiting Flow

One final effect related to the limits of flow that is unique to ECMO, specifically VV ECMO, is the concept of recirculation. Recirculation is an important concept in the management of VV ECMO that we will continue to discuss and review. In the current context, we will visit the implications of recirculation on the limits of flow.

Recirculation happens in VV ECMO, where blood is drained from the venous system and returned to the venous system. Ideally, deoxygenated blood is drained from the IVC, oxygenated, and then returned to the right atrium, where it can be returned to the body (Fig. 10.15).

Let's now zoom in and see what can happen as we increase blood flow (Fig. 10.16).

You can see that as we flow progressively higher, the drainage cannula exerts more of a negative pressure and eventually begins to pull oxygenated blood back into the circuit before it is circulated to the body. This has the effect of decreasing the effective blood flow. Any blood that is recirculated does not contribute to the oxygen delivery of the ECMO circuit, with the following relationship:

Effective blood flow = ECMO blood flow − recirculation

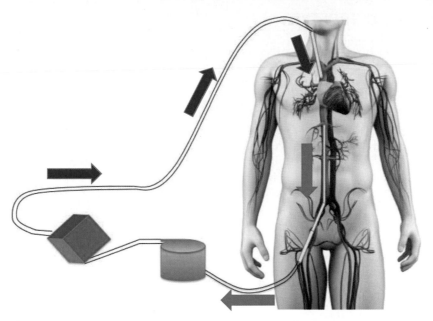

FIG. 10.15 Ideal ECMO blood delivery with drainage of deoxygenated blood and return of oxygenated blood. (Modified from SciePro/Shutterstock.com.)

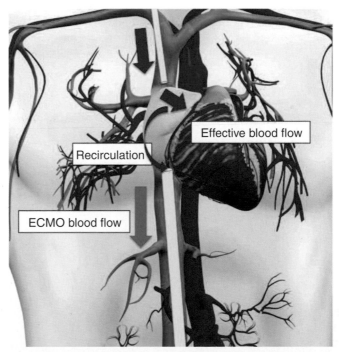

FIG. 10.16 The effect of recirculation on effective blood flow. (Modified from SciePro/Shutterstock.com.)

PUTTING IT ALL TOGETHER

Hopefully at the end of this chapter, you have a sense of flow, its role in oxygen delivery, and a grasp of the limitations to flow. There are many limitations to flow, and these should be carefully considered as flow is increased, decreased, or drops precipitously. Limits to flow play a large role in understanding how the ECMO blood flow is set. However, just because you are not limited in your flow does not necessarily mean that a certain flow should be maintained.

Rather, the titration of flow becomes a way to target the appropriate flow that matches both the capabilities of the circuit with the needs of the patient. We will continue to develop the tools needed to make this titration over the ensuing chapters, before diving more deeply into Flow Titration in Chapter 17. In the meantime, having a system to evaluate the circuit and assess its limitations like we have developed in this chapter is a significant step in the right direction.

SUGGESTED READING

Broman, L. M., Prahl Wittberg, L., Westlund, C. J., Gilbers, M., Perry da Câmara, L., & Westin, J. (2019). Pressure and flow properties of cannulae for extracorporeal membrane oxygenation II: drainage (venous) cannulae. *Perfusion*, *34*(1_suppl), 65–73.

Eckmann, D. M., Bowers, S., Stecker, M., & Cheung, A. T. (2000). Hematocrit, volume expander, temperature, and shear rate effects on blood viscosity. *Anesthesia & Analgesia*, *91*(3), 539–545.

Fernandez, K., Pyzdrowski, B., Schiller, D. W., & Smith, M. B. (2002). Understand the basics of centrifugal pump operation. *Chemical Engineering Progress*, *98*(5), 52–56.

Gajkowski, E. F., Herrera, G., Hatton, L., Velia Antonini, M., Vercaemst, L., & Cooley, E. (2022). ELSO guidelines for adult and pediatric extracorporeal membrane oxygenation circuits. *ASAIO Journal*, *68*(2), 133–152.

Galletti, P. M., Richardson, P. D., Snider, M. T., & Friedman, L. I. (1972). A standardized method for defining the overall gas transfer performance of artificial lungs. *ASAIO Journal*, *18*(1), 359–368.

Sirs, J. A. (1991). The flow of human blood through capillary tubes. *The Journal of Physiology*, *442*(1), 569–583.

11

Membrane Characteristics

Let's now turn our attention to the membrane itself. We will explore the function of the membrane oxygenator, its limits, and how we can appraise and assess this function at the bedside. Understanding the unique characteristics of the membrane is going to be essential – the better we understand the strengths and limitations of the membrane, the better we will be able to leverage its capabilities when we are treating our patients.

Specifically, we are going to explore the concept of sweep gas flow and how adjustments to the rate of flow lead to changes in CO_2. Recall the convention that we first introduced in the extracorporeal membrane oxygenation (ECMO) Fundamentals section on how to manipulate and adjust the ECMO circuit.

> FiO_2 and ECMO blood flow mainly affect **oxygenation/oxygen delivery** while sweep gas flow affects **ventilation/ CO_2 removal**

We spent the last chapter exploring the effect of blood flow on oxygen delivery. Now we will answer the following question:

Why does manipulation of sweep gas flow mainly affect CO_2 clearance?

Answering this question will require an exploration of the membrane itself and the ways that sweep gas flow interfaces with the membrane.

WHAT IS THE BASIC FUNCTION OF THE MEMBRANE OXYGENATOR?

Let's return to our illustration of the membrane at the most basic level. You will recall that blood flows into the membrane, diffusing around plastic tubes that carry gas, which establishes a semi-diffusible barrier between a sweep gas phase and a blood phase (Fig. 11.1).

Much like the alveolar-blood interface, this blood/gas interface does not allow the diffusion of blood components but is diffusible enough to allow oxygen and CO_2 to travel down their concentration gradients. That means that if the FiO_2 is set to 100%, the PaO_2 of the sweep gas flow would be around 713 mmHg while the PaO_2 of the venous blood flowing into the oxygenator is much lower, say around 40 mmHg. Therefore, O_2 flows down its concentration gradient, from an area of high concentration (sweep gas) to an area of low concentration (blood). Even if the blood has a relatively high oxygen content, with a PaO_2 of 55 mmHg or even 60 mmHg, the gradient between sweep gas and blood is so high that oxygen will still diffuse, such that the PaO_2 of the blood will increase.

In a similar manner, CO_2 will move in the opposite direction out of the blood, since it exists at a higher concentration in the venous blood, say around 45 mmHg, versus 0 mmHg in the sweep gas.

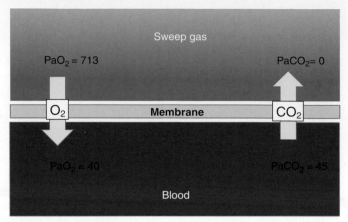

FIG. 11.1 The diffusion of O_2 and CO_2 across the membrane

With such large gradients existing between oxygen and CO_2 clearance, you can imagine that these gases are able to diffuse at high efficiencies.

IS ECMO MORE EFFICIENT AT OXYGENATION OR CO_2 CLEARANCE?

The answer here can be surprising. Many think oxygenation – it's called extracorporeal membrane *oxygenation* after all. Moreover, the relative gradient between PaO_2 in the sweep gas and in the blood is much greater. But the answer is CO_2 clearance. It's actually not even close – it is CO_2 clearance by a long shot. Why is that?

Efficiency of the Membrane: Effect of Relative Diffusibility

The main reason is diffusibility. CO_2 is more diffusible across the membrane. How much more diffusible? Six times more! This higher diffusibility allows for higher CO_2 clearance and overtakes the larger gradient that exists for oxygen between the sweep gas and blood.

Let's reflect on why this occurs. Imagine two lines at a toll booth to a bridge. One line is for cars with an automated pass. A sensor detects their pass and they can drive right through. The second line is for cars that have to pay cash. They have to stop, pay the operator, and receive change before proceeding on. If that first line is 6 times faster, it would not matter how many cars were in the second line; the concentration of cars from the first line on the bridge would be higher.

This is why sweep gas flow is so important to CO_2 clearance. The faster it flows, the more it clears CO_2 since CO_2 diffuses so much more rapidly.

Efficiency of CO_2 Clearance: Effect of Hemoglobin

The other reason that ECMO is so much more efficient at CO_2 clearance than oxygenation comes back to the difference between how oxygen is carried throughout the body and how CO_2 is carried throughout the body. You will no doubt recall from Chapter 1 that the way that oxygen is carried throughout the body is through binding to hemoglobin. This is for good reason – if it wasn't bound to hemoglobin, it would just diffuse to tissues based on proximity and there would be no efficient distribution throughout the body. Like we have established before – SaO_2 is more important to oxygen delivery than PaO_2.

CO_2 is different. It does not need to be delivered and distributed evenly like oxygen does. Which means that CO_2 can simply remain dissolved in the blood, represented by $PaCO_2$.

Now that we have established these premises, let's examine the effect of the membrane on oxygenation and CO_2 clearance.

Let's start with oxygenation. Say you have a normal venous saturation of 70% of the blood entering into the oxygenator. This may correspond to a PaO_2 of 40 mmHg, which is much lower than the PaO_2 of 713 mmHg in the sweep gas, allowing for excellent diffusion of O_2 into the blood, so much so that the PaO_2 of blood leaving the oxygenator is 400 mmHg with a saturation of 100% (Fig. 11.2).

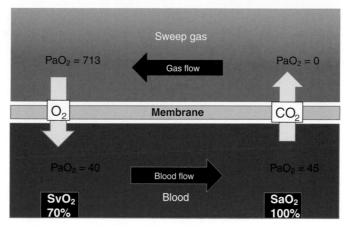

FIG. 11.2 The impact of hemoglobin saturation on membrane oxygen effectiveness

Now let's compare this to CO_2. In this case, the $PaCO_2$ of the blood entering into the oxygenator may be say 45 mmHg. This is significantly higher than the $PaCO_2$ of the sweep gas flow of 0 mmHg. Thus, the CO_2 molecules diffuse down their concentration gradient and the CO_2 is drawn down to <10 mmHg.

You can now see how CO_2 clearance can also be relatively more significant. Even though in this example, O_2 concentrations are increasing 10 fold and CO_2 concentrations are decreasing 10 fold, the parameter that matters to oxygen delivery of the body only increases by 30% (from 70% to 100%) (Fig. 11.3).

For oxygenation, you are limited by the saturation capacity of hemoglobin, while for CO_2 clearance, no such limit exists limiting $PaCO_2$.

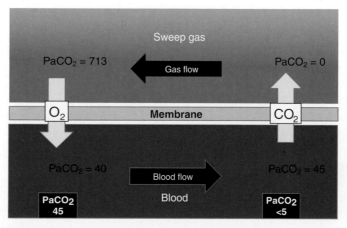

FIG. 11.3 The impact of dissolved CO_2 on membrane CO_2 clearance

LEVERAGING SWEEP GAS FLOW RATE

The sweep gas flow rate will allow for CO_2 to be swept away at a proportional rate. Therefore, the higher the rate of sweep gas flow, the higher the CO_2 clearance.

This works out in a favorable manner when it comes to how sweep is titrated. It means that the only limit to how high this gas rate can be increased is the capacity of the oxygenator/blender, which is usually 10–15 L/min.

Compare this to the limits of blood flow that we discussed in the prior chapter – everything from anatomic limitations to the limitations of the circuit/oxygenator to the preload dependence/afterload sensitivity of the pump to hemolysis to recirculation can limit blood flow. For sweep, it is a manner of turning a dial and increasing gas flow.

You can see that increasing sweep gas flow rates by 2–3× can easily be done, which cannot always be said about ECMO blood flow.

Does This Mean That Blood Flow Through the Membrane Has No Effect on CO_2 Clearance?

Blood flow actually can have a significant effect on CO_2 clearance. Higher blood flows translate into higher CO_2 clearance to a certain point, in a similar manner to how higher blood flow translates into higher oxygen delivery (Fig. 11.4).

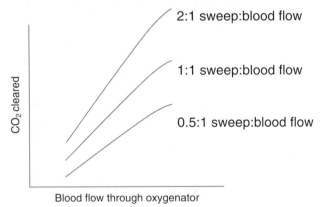

FIG. 11.4 CO_2 clearance as a function of sweep gas flow and blood flow

However, as compared to the oxygenation curve, this curve becomes steeper and accounts for more CO_2 clearance as the sweep gas flow increases compared to blood flow increases.

What does this mean clinically? Should we be targeting blood flow when we are attempting to optimize CO_2 clearance? Since sweep gas flow changes can be made so readily, my approach is to arrive at the ideal blood flow that is needed to meet oxygen delivery requirements and then adjust sweep gas flow accordingly to dial in the CO_2 clearance needs.

LIMITATIONS OF THE MEMBRANE OXYGENATOR

All of this assumes a normally functioning membrane oxygenator. An oxygenator can perform suboptimally for a number of reasons, from how blood is flowing to the function of its fibers. We will now dive deeper into the issues with membrane oxygenator function and review some of the patterns for assessing how the membrane loses effectiveness.

Effect of Thrombus Formation on the Function of Oxygenator

As time on ECMO increases, the performance and function of the oxygenator tends to decline. The primary reason for this decline involves the activation of a host of inflammatory and coagulation cascades as blood moves through the oxygenator. These cascades can lead to microscopic and larger clot formation on the fibers of the oxygenator that can literally disrupt the flow of gases across it (Figs. 11.5 and 11.6).

However, this process can often be quite unpredictable; some oxygenators can perform optimally for weeks to months, while others can last only a few days before showing signs of poor performance. This partially occurs due to variations in anticoagulation status, blood flow rates, and occurrence of disruptions in flow. However, there are likely a number of host factors that are not yet fully understood that also contribute to the upregulation of clot formation. We will discuss the regulation of the coagulation cascade in greater detail in Chapter 20.

Decreasing performance of the oxygenator due to clot formation can affect membrane function, alter the flow of blood, or cause damage to blood.

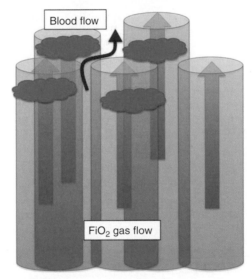

FIG. 11.5 Oxygenator thrombus formation

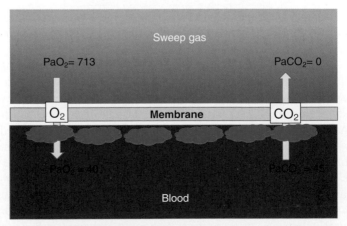

FIG. 11.6 Membrane oxygenator thrombus formation

EVALUATION OF OXYGENATOR FUNCTION

Evaluating the function of the oxygenator requires an assessment of the blood going in and out of the oxygenator. Often this comes in the form of assessing blood gases from three sources: the patient, pre-oxygenator, and post-oxygenator, as illustrated in Fig. 11.7.

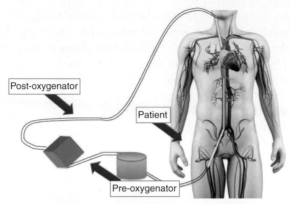

FIG. 11.7 Assessing oxygenator function with blood gas measurements: patient, pre-oxygenator, and post-oxygenator. (Modified from SciePro/Shutterstock.com.)

The reason for checking these gases is to give an adequate sense of the performance of the oxygenator and the clinical situation of what is going on with the patient.

1. Patient ABG: used to assess what is going on with the patient. Any changes to support, sweep gas flow, or blood flow are ultimately made to alter the parameters of this gas.
2. Post-oxygenator ABG: gives a sense of the performance of the oxygenator. The most important parameter is the PaO_2, but the $PaCO_2$ is also taken into consideration.
3. Pre-oxygenator: used for calibrating SvO_2 monitors, assessing for recirculation, approximating VO_2 (with limitation), and contextualizing CO_2 clearance.

Checking all three sources (known as "triple gases") is not necessary with every gas, but rather should be done if the desired effect is to examine both what is happening clinically with the patient and how the oxygenator is performing.

EVALUATION OF CO_2 CLEARANCE

CO_2 clearance (the difference in $PaCO_2$ pre-oxygenator and post-oxygenator) can give a sense of how the oxygenator is performing. Factors affecting CO_2 clearance include the $PaCO_2$ of the blood entering the oxygenator, the performance of the membrane, and the sweep gas flow rate. Thus, if $PaCO_2$ is relatively low entering the oxygenator, there may not be as much clearance of CO_2 since the $PaCO_2$ gradient between the blood and sweep gas is lower. Accordingly, if sweep gas flow is low, say because you are weaning down, the CO_2 clearance may be low. This is not due necessarily to a failing oxygenator, but rather due to a low rate of clearance due to the sweep gas flow rate.

As oxygenators start to have progressive thrombotic burden and a worsening performance, this can lead to a decreased diffusion of gases, which can manifest as a drop in CO_2 clearance.

Importantly, this decrease in CO_2 clearance may manifest before a drop in oxygenation. The high diffusibility of CO_2 under normal circumstances necessitates that a drop in the performance of the membrane may have a larger observable effect in CO_2 clearance. I start to consider oxygenator failure when the CO_2 clearance between pre-oxygenator and post-oxygenator is less than 10 mmHg despite being on a moderate amount of sweep (say 4–5 L/min).

EVALUATION OF OXYGENATION

Normally, PaO_2 is of less concern when we are evaluating blood gases, because saturation is the marker of adequate oxygen delivery. However, remember that the performance of the membrane oxygenator is dictated by how well gases can diffuse. Therefore, when evaluating the post-oxygenator gas, the PaO_2 is paramount, as it alone dictates how well the oxygenator is performing when it comes to allowing the diffusion of oxygen.

You should anticipate a high post-oxygenator PaO_2 if on 100% FiO_2 due to the high gradient that exists from the sweep gas (PaO_2 713 mmHg) to the blood (PaO_2 ~40 mmHg) (Fig. 11.8).

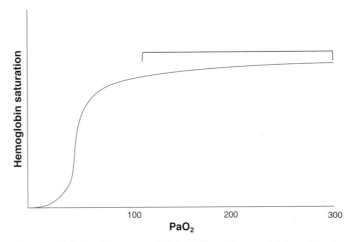

FIG. 11.8 Minimal impact of high PaO_2 on hemoglobin saturation

Additionally, as you may recall from our hemoglobin dissociation curve there is a flat portion of the curve where PaO_2 increases but has a negligible effect on saturation. Although this PaO_2 does not improve the delivery of oxygen significantly, monitoring for changes in the PaO_2, say from 450 to 200 over the course of a couple of days, may be a significant indicator that the oxygenator function is worsening, even if the saturation of the blood leaving the oxygenator remains at 100%.

EVALUATION OF MEMBRANE FUNCTION: DAMAGE TO BLOOD CELLS/CONSUMPTION

An important part of the evaluation of the function of the oxygenator is the effect on the blood itself. As clot burden increases, these clots can exert a host of adverse effects on the blood that is circulating through the membrane.

One such effect is damage to the cells itself, primarily red blood cells. Close evaluation for markers of hemolysis (jaundice, elevated plasma-free hemoglobin, elevated lactate dehydrogenase (LDH), elevated bilirubin, and dark urine) can help to identify worsening oxygenator function, particularly if revolutions per minute (RPMs) to the pump have remained relatively stable.

Thrombus and clot formation can have the additional adverse effect of upregulating more clot formation, therefore exerting a consumptive effect of the membrane. In this case, there may be a consumptive coagulopathy with a drop in fibrinogen, coagulation parameters, and platelets similar to disseminated intravascular coagulation (DIC) but occurring within the oxygenator rather than intravascularly.

Evidence of any of these phenomena point toward a worsening oxygenator function, even in the presence of adequate gas exchange, and is thus often part of the daily evaluation of the circuit.

EVALUATION OF MEMBRANE FUNCTION: EFFECT ON MEMBRANE BLOOD FLOW AND PRESSURE

The third manifestation of a failing membrane is a change in pressure and blood flow. This is largely due to thrombus formation on the oxygenator, which impedes flow by adding afterload to the pump. The added afterload decreases the pressure differential that the pump is able to generate, and eventually leads to a drop in flows. This drop can be gradual or precipitous. Usually, alteration in pressures is a late manifestation of oxygenator failure, but it can happen right after cannulation, likely due to the effect of an existing thrombus that gets sucked into the oxygenator by the drainage cannula.

If pressures are being measured/transduced, then transmembrane pressures measured pre-oxygenator and post-oxygenator can help to identify oxygenator thrombus and worsening function.

To review our process for evaluating membrane pressures, we can measure circuit pre-oxygenator, post-oxygenator, and pre-pump (if you have an integrated sensor). The highest pressure of the circuit will be the pressure directly after the pump (pre-oxygenator), as this is the highest pressure that will be generated in the circuit. After this, the pressure drops across the membrane, to a degree that is equal to the transmembrane pressure or delta P. The pressure post-oxygenator then drops gradually until it equals the mean arterial pressure (MAP) or central venous pressure (CVP), depending on if you are on VA or VV ECMO (Fig. 11.9).

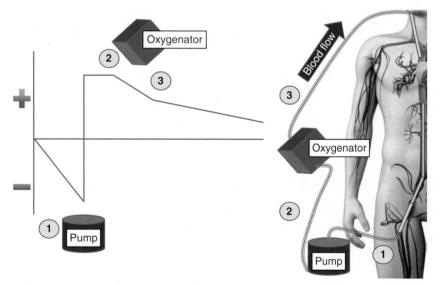

FIG. 11.9 Pressures throughout the ECMO circuit. (Modified from SciePro/Shutterstock.com.)

We can now contrast this to the below situation, where there is a thrombus formation on the oxygenator. In this case, the pressure needed to maintain adequate flow rises precipitously, otherwise you would experience a drop in flows. You will note that the pressure at position 3 (post-oxygenator) remains the same; the escalation in delta P results from an increase in pre-oxygenator pressure due to the obstruction across the oxygenator (Fig. 11.10).

Escalation in membrane pressures, especially rapid escalation over the course of minutes to hours, should be intervened on rapidly as this can be a harbinger of impending circuit failure.

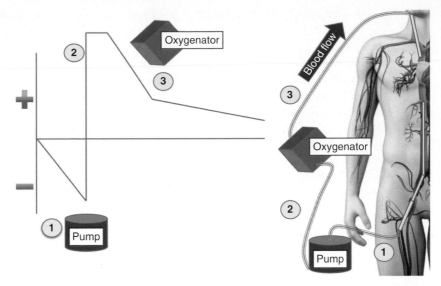

FIG. 11.10 Impact of oxygenator thrombus with elevated post-pump/pre-oxygenator pressure. (Modified from SciePro/Shutterstock.com.)

FAILURE OF MEMBRANE FUNCTION DUE TO RECIRCULATION

Let's return to the concept of recirculation and explore its implications for affecting membrane function. As you'll remember, recirculation is a circumstance unique to VV ECMO, which involves blood that is being returned from the circuit being sucked back into the circuit before it has the opportunity to be circulated to the rest of the body (Fig. 11.11).

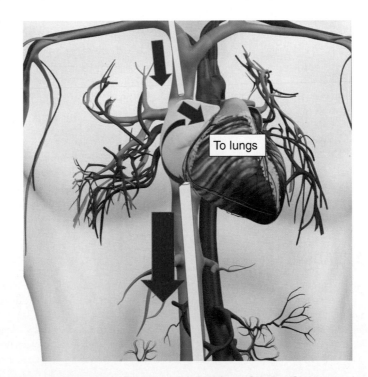

FIG. 11.11 Recirculation of blood. (Modified from SciePro/Shutterstock.com.)

You will recall that the first adverse effect of recirculation is a decrease in effective blood flow, since any volume of blood that is recirculated is simply going back to the circuit and not being distributed to the body.

The causes of recirculation are as follows:

1. Excessive blood flow rates: the high negative pressures required to maintain these flows exert more pull on returning blood.
2. Cannula malposition: lack of adequate space between the return and the drainage cannula can allow for returned blood to get sucked back into the drainage cannula.
3. High negative intrathoracic pressures: coughing or deep breathing, with strong exertion of the diaphragm, can lead to a negative pressure causing recirculation either continuously or rhythmically, with an increase in recirculation with each breath.
4. Right ventricular failure: due to returned blood not being adequately circulated into the pulmonary circulation, backing up, and then being sucked into the drainage cannula

How Does Recirculation Adversely Affect Membrane Function?

Recirculation also affects membrane function, rendering it less effective. Let's consider an example to illustrate.

Your patient is on VV ECMO. You are flowing 3 L, with a venous saturation of 60% and a patient saturation of 90%. Hoping to improve the saturation, a well-meaning member of the staff increases the blood flow to 5 L. The saturation decreased to 85% and the venous saturation increased to 80%.

What happened here? Why did the saturation go *down*?

This example illustrates the two adverse effects of recirculation. The first is that the effective flow went down, as the higher blood flow pulled more blood into the drainage cannula, and less was able to flow to the patient.

The second is how recirculation decreases the effectiveness of the membrane. Prior to going up on flow, the membrane was able to raise the saturation of the patient 30%, from 60% to 90%. But raising the saturation of the drained blood decreases the amount that the membrane can oxygenate, which is now only 5%.

> Recirculation adversely affects the patient by decreasing the effective blood flow **and** by decreasing the effective function of the membrane.

PUTTING IT TOGETHER

Understanding the membrane function is an essential component of understanding the physiology of ECMO support. Like most aspects of ECMO, membrane function requires serial attention to trends. Evidence of membrane failure can be more readily recognized when placed into the context of what is happening with the patient on a daily basis.

SUGGESTED READING

Ficial, B., Vasques, F., Zhang, J., Whebell, S., Slattery, M., & Lamas, T. (2021). Physiological basis of extracorporeal membrane oxygenation and extracorporeal carbon dioxide removal in respiratory failure. *Membranes, 11*(3), 225.

Bishoy, Z., Sheldrake, J., & Pellegrino, V. (2020). Extracorporeal membrane oxygenation and V/Q ratios: an ex vivo analysis of CO2 clearance within the Maquet Quadrox-iD oxygenator. *Perfusion, 35*(1_suppl), 29–33.

Horton, S., Thuys, C., Bennett, M., Augustin, S., Rosenberg, M., & Brizard, C. (2004). Experience with the Jostra Rotaflow and QuadroxD oxygenator for ECMO. *Perfusion, 19*(1), 17–23.

Sun, L., Kaesler, A., Fernando, P., Thompson, A. J., Toomasian, J. M., & Bartlett, R. H. (2018). CO_2 clearance by membrane lungs. *Perfusion, 33*(4), 249–253.

Chung, M., Shiloh, A. L., & Carlese, A. (2014). Monitoring of the adult patient on venoarterial extracorporeal membrane oxygenation. *The Scientific World Journal, 2014*, 393258.

Broman, M., Frenckner, B., Bjällmark, A., & Broomé, M. (2015). Recirculation during veno-venous extracorporeal membrane oxygenation–a simulation study. *The International Journal of Artificial Organs, 38*(1), 23–30.

Yeager, T., & Roy, S. (2017). Evolution of gas permeable membranes for extracorporeal membrane oxygenation. *Artificial Organs, 41*(8), 700–709.

12

Veno-Venous ECMO Physiology

Now we are at the point where we can start to apply our discussion of physiology to specific extra-corporeal membrane oxygenation (ECMO) configurations. As you will see, even though they both use the same pump, circuit, membrane oxygenator, and cannulas, our two flavors of ECMO, veno-venous ECMO and veno-arterial ECMO, provide very different, support. You will get a sense of the subtleties related to these modalities in the chapters to follow.

In this chapter, we will focus on veno-venous ECMO, otherwise known as respiratory ECMO or VV ECMO.

VV ECMO: THE BASICS

Let's start this discussion by reminding ourselves of the configuration of VV ECMO. When we refer to VV ECMO, we are draining deoxygenated blood from the venous system, running it through our membrane oxygenator, and returning the oxygenated blood to the venous circulation where it gets circulated to the body through the native right ventricle (Fig. 12.1).

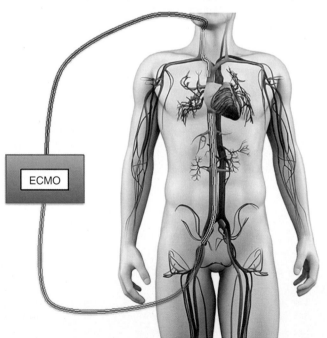

FIG. 12.1 Veno-venous ECMO. (Modified from SciePro/Shutterstock.com.)

The mechanism allows for improvement of oxygenation and ventilation/CO_2 removal parameters in patients with respiratory failure. We will further our understanding of this mechanism and physiology, exploring the rationale for the beneficial and the potential adverse hemodynamic and respiratory effects of VV ECMO.

MECHANISM OF HEMODYNAMIC/RESPIRATORY BENEFITS OF VV ECMO

Let's start by reviewing the physiologic rationale for VV ECMO. Remember that ECMO does not cure any of the inciting etiologies. Rather, it is only effective to the extent that it mitigates the toxicity related to the support that is required in response to an insult. Thus, even if the physiologic rationale is intriguing, it is only relevant in as much as it translates to an improvement in the outcome of the patient.

With that in mind, we will now explore the two primary mechanisms of benefit related to VV ECMO support, improvement of shunt and improvement of right ventricular hemodynamics.

Let's review each.

EFFECT OF VV ECMO ON SHUNT PHYSIOLOGY

As discussed in Chapter 4, while there are a variety of mechanisms for hypoxia (hypoventilation, diffusion defect, low inspired oxygen levels, intracardiac shunt), shunt physiology plays an important role. When there is worsening mismatch at the alveolar/blood vessel interface leading to V/Q of less than 1, blood shunts across the pulmonary circulation without participating in gas exchange (Fig. 12.2).

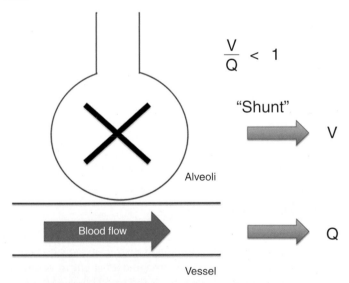

FIG. 12.2 Shunt physiology as a cause of hypoxia

This is especially important because as the percentage of shunt increases, the lungs become less responsive to administration of supplemental oxygen, and positive pressure is required to decrease the shunted alveoli.

The effect of positive pressure is relevant to our discussion with ECMO because as respiratory failure worsens, the increasing shunt and decreasing pulmonary compliance combines to require escalating ventilator pressures, and worsens the potential for damage to the lungs due to the ventilator in the form of barotrauma/volutrauma.

Shunt in VV ECMO behaves much differently.

In this case, even though blood is still being shunted across the pulmonary circulation without participating in gas exchange in the lungs, some of this blood is now already oxygenated from the ECMO circuit, and the shunted blood is oxygenated (Fig. 12.3).

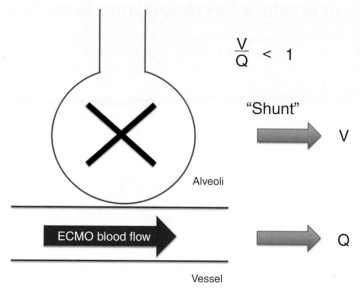

$$\frac{V}{Q} < 1$$

"Shunt"

V

Alveoli

ECMO blood flow

Q

Vessel

FIG. 12.3 The effect of shunt in VV ECMO

The result is that shunt fraction is improved even if V:Q matching is not. In fact, VV ECMO may even worsen V:Q matching by decreasing hypoxic vasoconstriction and increasing perfusion to damaged potions of the lungs.

This may seem like an esoteric point. You may be asking – why is this important to the patient?

Since shunt fraction is less of a priority while on ECMO, you do not need to improve shunt fraction with higher and potentially damaging airway pressures.

The extent that you can reduce elevated/damaging ventilator pressures/volumes with ECMO will determine the extent that it is able to benefit your patient.

HEMODYNAMIC EFFECTS OF VV ECMO

To better understand the hemodynamic effects of VV ECMO, let's start with the hemodynamic effects of hypoxia. If oxygen levels precipitously drop, how does this affect the cardiac output and blood pressure? To help answer, let's imagine a patient in respiratory failure who has a cardiac arrest due to a respiratory arrest. What is the typical presentation?

Usually, if you were to review the telemetry and monitor, the presentation is sinus rhythm, followed by a bradycardia, followed by hypotension, followed by arrest. Why this pattern?

The answer is that hypoxia causes hypoxic vasoconstriction as an adaptive mechanism to overcome V/Q mismatch. This vasoconstriction raises right ventricular afterload, which will drop right ventricular output leading to conduction abnormalities (bradycardia) followed by cessation of right ventricular output altogether (arrest).

You may also recall from Chapter 2 the other causes of elevated pulmonary vascular constriction that can worsen right ventricular afterload and precipitate right heart failure:

$\downarrow O_2$
$\downarrow pH$
$\downarrow$ temperature
$\downarrow$ pulmonary compliance
$\uparrow CO_2$
$\uparrow \alpha$-adrenergic tone

Now let's return to what happens during VV ECMO – where blood is returned to the right atrium with high levels of O_2, low levels of CO_2, and is temperature controlled. The effect can be a rapid improvement in hemodynamics as the oxygenated blood reduces pulmonary vasoconstriction, decreases right ventricular afterload and eventually increases right ventricular output, leading to improved left ventricular filling, and improvement in overall cardiac output.

This hemodynamic effect of VV ECMO can lead to an improvement in DO_2 that is just as significant as the infusion of oxygenated blood via the circuit.

The degree that VV ECMO improves hemodynamics depends on the degree to which cardiac output is limited by right ventricular afterload due to hypoxia/hypercapnea. Persistent hypotension following initiation of VV ECMO should raise suspicion and prompt investigation for other causes of shock, namely vasodilation and sepsis.

It is difficult to predict the hemodynamic effect on right ventricular cardiac output that can be anticipated from the initiation of VV ECMO. At this point, it is important to be aware of the potential for improvement and to factor the anticipation of this improvement into the prediction of how ECMO will improve the patient with hypoxic respiratory failure. Understanding the physiology behind patients who respond and those who do not respond will be an essential part of selection for ECMO as well as management while on ECMO.

This is a nuanced way of thinking about VV ECMO support, but will ultimately equip you with a better sense of our sweet spot (patients who will do well with ECMO who would do poorly without ECMO) rather than just selecting patients based on specific respiratory parameters (P:F, OI, ventilator requirements, etc.).

Mechanism of Adverse Respiratory/Hemodynamic Effect on VV ECMO

When considering ECMO and the physiologic effects of ECMO we must always consider the harmful effect of ECMO support. Usually we do this by thinking about the adverse events that are often reported for ECMO – bleeding, clotting, stroke, damage to underlying structures. However, we should also consider the physiologic risks of support, particularly what limits the effectiveness of support and the degree of toxicity of conventional support that may need to be incorporated into the care as a result.

Limitations to the Respiratory Effects of VV ECMO

Said another way, what are the physiologic mechanisms behind hypoxia for patients on VV ECMO.

Wait, hypoxia on VV ECMO?

You read that right. Although VV ECMO is designed to mitigate hypoxia, hypoxia can be quite common. Let's explore why.

For a patient who is not on ECMO, as the lungs become progressively more compromised, and shunt is increasing despite all interventions, you can anticipate more blood to be shunted across the lungs, such that the saturation of blood entering the left atrium approximates the saturation of the blood leaving the right ventricle (Fig. 12.4).

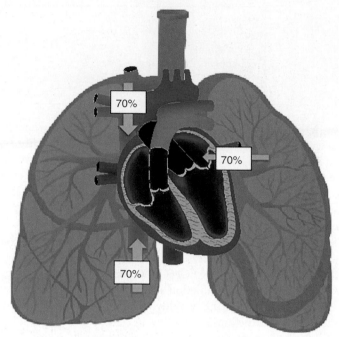

FIG. 12.4 As shunt increases, the saturation of blood returning to the left heart from the lungs approximates the SvO_2. (Modified from YanGe_Tam/Shutterstock.com.)

This will then lead to a decrease in the saturation of the venous blood returning to the heart, which in turn drops the saturation of the blood returning from the lungs, leading to a rapid deterioration.

ECMO can mitigate this downward spiral by draining the venous blood that would be going across the shunted pulmonary blood vessels and replacing it with oxygenated blood. To the extent that the drainage/return of this blood is greater than the native cardiac output, this will result in a patient oxygen saturation of 100% (Fig. 12.5).

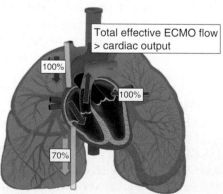

FIG. 12.5 The effect of shunt on ECMO when ECMO blood flow is higher than cardiac output. (Modified from YanGe_Tam/Shutterstock.com.)

However, let's consider this same clinical situation, except now, where the native cardiac output picks up and is greater than the ECMO blood flow by a factor of 2:1 (with a right ventricular output say of 8 L compared to a maximum effective achievable ECMO blood flow of 4 L). In this case, half of the blood that is being circulated across the shunted pulmonary circulation is 100% oxygenated while the other half is shunted venous blood that is 70% saturated.

In this case, the expected saturation of blood returning to the left heart and consequently the expected patient saturation would be 85%, the average between the blood returning from the oxygenator (100% saturated) and the blood that is not flowing through the oxygenator (70% saturated) (Fig. 12.6).

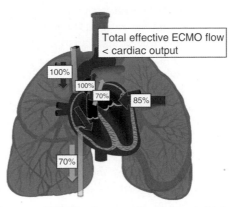

FIG. 12.6 The effect of shunt on ECMO when cardiac output is higher than ECMO blood flow. (Modified from YanGe_Tam/Shutterstock.com.)

Continuing this thought experiment, as the ratio of cardiac output to achievable ECMO blood flow continues to increase, the percentage of deoxygenated blood returning to the left heart increases, such that the patient saturation starts to approximate the saturation of the venous blood (70% in this case).

OTHER VARIABLES CONTRIBUTING TO OXYGENATION IN VV ECMO

What this example is describing is a relationship between two competing circulations: the native circulation/lungs and the ECMO circulation/membrane oxygenator. The greater the contribution of the native circulation, the more the saturation of the patient will approximate the saturation of what the lungs can contribute outside of ECMO (SaO_2 native lungs). If we were to write this relationship as an equation, it might look something like this:

$$SaO_{2\,patient} = SaO_{2\,oxygenator} \left[\frac{\text{Effective ECMO flow}}{\text{Cardiac output}} \right]$$

$$+ SaO_{2\,native\,lungs} \left[\frac{\text{Cardiac output} - \text{Effective ECMO flow}}{\text{Cardiac output}} \right]$$

This is the central equation for understanding hypoxia on VV ECMO. The more you can understand the concepts behind this equation, the better you will have a system to troubleshoot hypoxia. Let's evaluate each component.

SaO$_2$ of the Oxygenator

This is the saturation of the blood returning from the oxygenator. Assuming a working membrane oxygenator, this can be assumed to be 100%.

Effective ECMO Flow

> Effective ECMO flow = ECMO blood flow − recirculation

Remember we say effective ECMO flow, not blood flow. Effective ECMO flow is the blood flow that is actually reaching the patient. It combines the limits of the circuit/pump that were described in Chapter 10 as well as recirculation. Recirculation decreases the effective ECMO flow according to the following equation:

The challenging thing about recirculation is that it can't be quantified, only inferred/estimated based on blood gases. Recirculation should be a consideration anytime there is less than a 20% difference between the pre-oxygenator blood gas and the patient arterial blood gas.

Cardiac Output

As cardiac output (specifically right ventricular output) increases, the proportion of blood going across the lungs increases. The higher the native cardiac output compared to the effective ECMO blood flow, the closer the patient saturation will be to the native lung SaO$_2$.

Does dropping the cardiac output make sense? It is possible that lowering cardiac output (say with beta blockade) will result in an increased SaO$_2$. However, this higher SaO$_2$ may not contribute to a higher DO$_2$, since you had to trade off cardiac output to get it.

When does decreasing cardiac output make sense? When the elevated heart rate/stroke volume is not a function of the body trying to augment DO$_2$ – fever, pain, agitation, hypermetabolic state, excess pressors, etc. In these cases, bringing down heart rate/cardiac output may have the effect of treating the underlying cause and improving saturations.

SaO$_2$ Native Lungs

This is the saturation that would be returning to the left atrium if the ECMO circuit was not running. It is comprised of two variables:
1. Contribution of the lungs
2. Native venous oxygen saturation: function of DO$_2$:VO$_2$

Application of This Equation

This equation demonstrates the essential points but doesn't require actual calculations at the bedside. Rather than trying to calculate numbers, use this equation to structure your approach and infer what is going on with the patient. Let's use an example.

Say you are taking care of the following patient:

44 year old man on day 3 of VV ECMO (cannulated by femoral-internal jugular vein approach)

Blood flow 3.5 L, 1800 RPM, sweep gas flow 3 L, FiO$_2$ 100%

Ventilator: AC/VC, 70% FiO$_2$, TV 300 mL, PEEP 10, rate 20

ABG: 7.39, 41, PaO$_2$ 45, **SaO$_2$ 75%**

If we want to improve this saturation, there are only a few options.

1. **Increase effective ECMO blood flow.** Limitations of this strategy include limits of the pump, oxygenator, resistance of the circuit, effects of RPM (hemolysis), and recirculation.

If blood flow is increased, attention should be paid to excessive circuit pressures, evidence of hemolysis (LDH, hemolysis, dark urine), and evidence of recirculation (elevation of pre-oxygenator SvO_2).

2. **Decrease cardiac output**. Can consider but this may not help DO_2. Attention should be paid to evidence of worsening DO_2:VO_2 ratio (such as decreased SvO_2, lactic acidosis, or decreased urine output).

3. **Increase SaO_2 of native lungs**. This can be done through augmentation of the mechanical ventilation settings or augmentation of native DO_2:VO_2. Higher ventilator settings may risk toxicity of the ventilator. Since DO_2 is function of SaO_2, cardiac output, and hemoglobin, this comes in the form of administration of blood.

Now you are in a position to compare the competing circulations (ECMO v. native) and to evaluate the effect of your interventions. Consider the following stepwise approach to the patient with hypoxia on VV ECMO in Fig. 12.7.

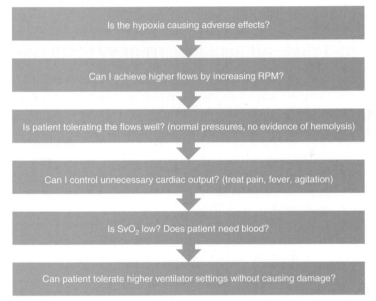

FIG. 12.7 Stepwise approach to the patient with hypoxia on VV ECMO. *RPM*, Revolutions per minute.

You can see how you are now adopting a much more nuanced approach than only increasing the ventilator or worse, doing everything at once with no ability to evaluate the effect and understand the physiology of what is going on with the patient.

LIMITATIONS TO THE CARDIAC/HEMODYNAMIC EFFECTS OF VV ECMO

Recall the hemodynamic rationale for VV ECMO is improvement of right ventricular afterload, through decrease in hypoxia/hypercapneia-mediated vasoconstriction. However, right ventricular failure can be common in VV ECMO, even with optimization of O_2/CO_2 levels.

The likely etiology of right ventricular failure/elevated pulmonary pressures in VV ECMO is vasoconstriction due to damaged lung that is mediated by cell-mediated/inflammatory mechanisms and poor pulmonary compliance. It is possible that this allows for improvement of V/Q matching in the presence of chronic hypoxia. In these cases, simply correcting O_2/CO_2 levels of the blood circulating to the pulmonary circulation does not improve the right ventricular afterload or function.

Rather, VV ECMO flow may serve to make this right ventricular function worse. In chronic pulmonary hypertension due to lung disease, elevated right ventricular afterload due to chronic hypoxia decreases overall cardiac output leading to an adaptive drop in filling pressures. By contrast, in a patient on VV ECMO, when the right ventricle fails due to worsening pulmonary disease/inflammatory mediators, there is no drop in filling pressures, as the flow of blood returning from the ECMO circuit remains constant.

The effect of a failing right ventricle on VV ECMO is less effective ECMO function. This happens in the following ways:

1. Worsening right ventricular output, with less ECMO blood flow circulating to the systemic circulation
2. Higher right ventricular filling pressures, with eventual worsening of right ventricular systolic function as well as left ventricular systolic function due to ventricular interdependence (see Chapter 2)
3. Less blood that is able to go forward past the right ventricle, leading to increasing recirculation and decreased effective ECMO blood flow

PUTTING IT TOGETHER: THE RISK-BENEFIT OF VV ECMO SUPPORT

We have spent a lot of time in this chapter discovering the rationale and limitations of VV ECMO support. This is not just a theoretical exercise, but rather a description of the physiologic subtypes of patients who do well with VV ECMO and patients in whom the benefits of VV ECMO are limited.

In all cases, there is a risk-benefit of ECMO support that must be considered. There are limitations to ECMO support as well as adverse effects. Just as we have explored the dose-related response of conventional care when it comes to vasopressors, fluids, and ventilation support, there is a dose-related response to ECMO support. This exists in terms of blood flow, duration of support, and hemodynamic effects.

We can conceptualize the overall risk profile of ECMO support as illustrated in Fig. 12.8, imagining a clinical improvement that exists to a point, after which, harmful effects of increasing blood flow take over, and there is a point of diminishing returns.

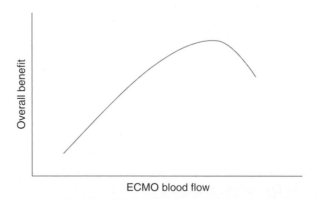

FIG. 12.8 ECMO blood flow risk-benefit

The decision about whether ECMO support should be titrated up or down needs to be put into the context of the benefit and harm, and can be elucidated by attention to the response to any changes.

SUGGESTED READING

Darryl, A., Bacchetta, M., & Brodie., D. (2015). Recirculation in venovenous extracorporeal membrane oxygenation. *ASAIO Journal*, *61*(2), 115–121.

Grant, C., Jr. (2021). ECMO and right ventricular failure: review of the literature. *Journal of Intensive Care Medicine*, *36*(3), 352–360.

Montisci, A., Maj, G., Zangrillo, A., Winterton, D., & Pappalardo, F. (2015). Management of refractory hypoxemia during venovenous extracorporeal membrane oxygenation for ARDS. *ASAIO Journal*, *61*(3), 227–236.

Patel, B., Arcaro, M., & Chatterjee, S. (2019). Bedside troubleshooting during venovenous extracorporeal membrane oxygenation (ECMO). *Journal of Thoracic Disease*, *11*(Suppl 14), S1698.

13

Veno-Arterial ECMO Physiology

Let's now move our discussion to the physiology of veno-arterial extracorporeal membrane oxygenation (VA ECMO). As you will come to appreciate, VA ECMO is a very different type of support than veno-venous extracorporeal membrane oxygenation (VV ECMO). These next few chapters will equip you with a much better sense of some of the subtleties related to this mode.

Similar to VV ECMO, VA ECMO involves a drainage cannula in the venous system. The blood is run through the same blood pump, membrane oxygenator, and circuit. However, the return cannula is implanted into the arterial system. As opposed to VV ECMO, which was dependent on the native cardiac output, the blood flow for VA ECMO translates to some of the overall cardiac output (Fig. 13.1).

There are limitations and rationale to the use of VA ECMO support. Let's start to contextualize these by introducing the vicious cycle of cardiogenic shock.

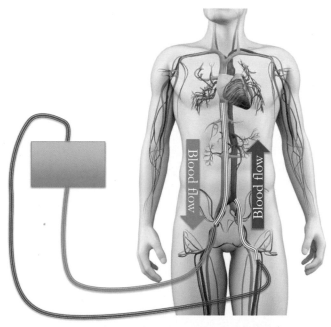

FIG. 13.1 Veno-arterial ECMO. (Modified from SciePro/Shutterstock.com.)

VICIOUS CYCLE OF CARDIOGENIC SHOCK

Cardiogenic shock can be one of the most devastating forms of shock, with mortality that can be as high as 85%. Worse yet, it is rapid, with a large proportion of patients dying within hours. You can see why we spent so much time talking about recognition, diagnosis, and identification of shock in the Physiology section. You will see that the reason for the rapid and devastating manifestation is the vicious cycle that is triggered.

The usual way of thinking is that decreased cardiac output leads to decreased perfusion, which leads to decompensation (Fig. 13.2)

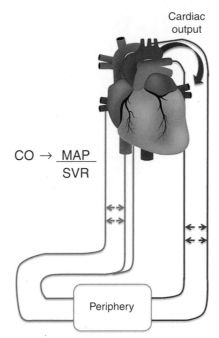

$$CO \rightarrow \frac{MAP}{SVR}$$

FIG. 13.2 Decreased cardiac output leading to decreased overall perfusion. *MAP*, Mean arterial pressure; *SVR*, systemic vascular resistance. (Modified from Ody_Stocker/Shutterstock.com.)

While this is true, there is much more at play here, with multiple mechanisms of decompensation that re-inforce and compound each other. Let's explore some of these effects.

Decreased Cardiac Output

Cardiac output is the driver of perfusion pressure, which is ultimately required for the forward flow of blood and delivery of oxygen. An insult to the cardiac function, whether ischemic due to myocardial ischemia, inflammatory as in myocarditis, obstructive as in pulmonary embolism or tamponade, or structural as in valvular/septal rupture, ultimately leads to a drop in cardiac output. As this output drops, the pressure head required to drive the forward flow of blood becomes progressively difficult to maintain, leading to a compensation in systemic vascular resistance (SVR) to maintain the forward flow of blood.

Decreased Coronary Perfusion

A drop in blood pressure affects the perfusion of all organs, but a decrease to the coronary blood vessels can be especially devastating because it serves to further worsen myocardial ischemia and further drop cardiac output.

Increased Left Ventricular End Diastolic Pressures (LVEDP)

Elevated SVR maintains the pressure needed to drive the forward flow of blood, much like putting your thumb over a hose may allow water to reach further if the flow of water decreases. However, this comes at a price – worsening afterload. As afterload increases, the left ventricular output starts to fall, which leads to less blood ejected with each heartbeat, and increasing the blood that remains in the ventricular cavity at the end of diastole (Fig. 13.3).

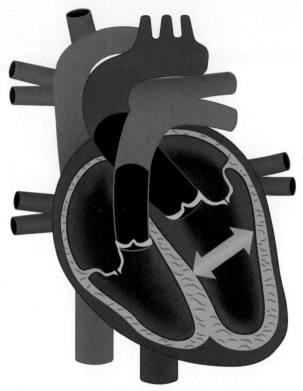

FIG. 13.3 Effect of afterload on failing left ventricle leading to increased left ventricular end diastolic pressure. (Modified from Ody_Stocker/Shutterstock.com.)

This elevated pressure has several adverse effects, especially in a failing and potentially ischemic left ventricle:

- Higher pressures can compress cardiac muscle causing wall stress leading to worsening ischemia
- Higher left ventricular pressures can exert higher pressures on blood returning from the lungs which can lead to pulmonary edema
- Pulmonary edema can lead to further hypoxia worsening overall oxygen delivery to the heart tissue which can further drop the cardiac output

You can see how this contributes to a downward spiral, with one adverse effect compounding on another.

Acidosis

As oxygen delivery worsens in the setting of hypoxia and decreased cardiac output, the cells throughout the body have less available oxygen to carry out aerobic metabolism. This causes them to shift to anaerobic metabolism, with worsening acidosis ensuing. While this process temporarily allows for the generation of energy at the cellular level, acidosis can precipitate vasodilation, worsening both venous return and shock.

Acute Kidney Injury

Amongst the first organs affected by worsening shock and oxygen delivery are the kidneys. The response can be adaptive initially, causing fluid retention and improvement in preload, but injury can ensue, leading to further fluid retention and decreased clearance. This can worsen acidosis and lead to volume overload with a host of adverse effect to include worsening pulmonary edema.

Right Ventricular Distension

The other adverse effect of volume overload is right ventricular distension. Remember that preload only helps the right ventricle to a point, after which there is little more stretch that can be accommodated by the less muscular ventricle. Further increase in right ventricular filling pressures can cause a precipitous decline in the output of the failing right ventricle and can decrease left ventricular output as the distended right ventricle begins to compress on the left ventricle (Fig. 13.4).

This can worsen if excessive fluids are administered to counteract the shock in this case.

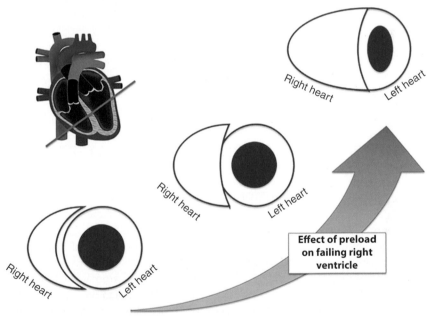

FIG. 13.4 The adverse effect of escalating preload on a failing right ventricle. (Modified from Ody_Stocker/Shutterstock.com.)

Increased Right Ventricular Afterload

The right ventricle is very afterload sensitive and will worsen in the following scenarios: hypoxia, hypercapnia, acidosis, hypothermia, decreased pulmonary compliance, and excessive pressor administration. As shock and pulmonary edema progress, all of these combine to worsen the pulmonary pressures and resistance that the right ventricle must work against, further decreasing output.

Summary of Vicious Cycle of Cardiogenic Shock

When taken together, we can see how these components of the vicious cycle of cardiogenic shock can compound on each other leading to a rapid decompensation. Although these components can all seem destructive, by separating out into their components we can have a better approach to all that is going on with a patient in cardiogenic shock, give a better framework to assess the overall effect of interventions, and define the role of mechanical circulatory support such as ECMO (Fig. 13.5)

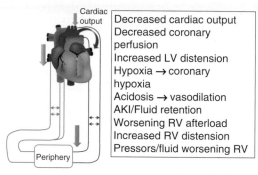

FIG. 13.5 Vicious cycle of cardiogenic shock. *AKI,* Acute kidney injury; *LV,* left ventricular; *RV,* right ventricular. (Modified from Ody_Stocker/Shutterstock.com.)

RATIONALE OF VA ECMO IN CARDIOGENIC SHOCK: EFFECT ON THE VICIOUS CYCLE

Let's now introduce VA ECMO and define how it is going to interact with this vicious cycle. There are two flavors of VA ECMO, central VA ECMO, where the cannulas are inserted directly onto the great blood vessels/heart, and peripheral VA ECMO, where the cannulas are inserted into the femoral blood vessels. We will discuss the physiology of central VA ECMO in Chapter 15, so for this chapter, we will focus on peripheral VA ECMO.

The blood flow is unique in VA ECMO, differing from VV ECMO in that blood is drained out of the venous system via a drainage cannula implanted into the inferior vena cava (IVC), and returned into the arterial system in a retrograde fashion against the normal flow of blood (Fig. 13.6).

The dynamics of this blood flow pattern are unique. Let's explore the effects this may have in the context of cardiogenic shock.

Effect #1: Support MAP

The effect of blood flow in ECMO is profound. In contrast to VV ECMO, where ECMO oxygen delivery is dependent on the native cardiac output, it is additive in VA ECMO, such that the total cardiac output is the summation of the native cardiac output and the ECMO blood flow (Fig. 13.7)

Since cardiac output is the mean arterial pressure (MAP)/SVR, an increase in overall output/perfusion translates into a higher MAP, or, importantly, allows for a decrease in SVR.

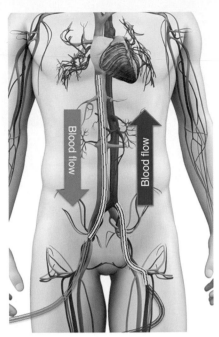

FIG. 13.6 Schematic of blood flow in peripheral VA ECMO. (Modified from SciePro/Shutterstock.com.)

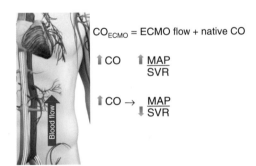

CO_{ECMO} = ECMO flow + native CO

$\uparrow CO \quad \uparrow \dfrac{MAP}{SVR}$

$\uparrow CO \rightarrow \dfrac{MAP}{\downarrow SVR}$

FIG. 13.7 Impact of VA ECMO flow on overall perfusion pressure and systemic vascular resistance. (Modified from SciePro/Shutterstock.com.)

Effect #2: Decrease SVR

Maintaining an adequate MAP at a lower SVR is essential. The whole purpose of MAP is to maintain the pressure needed to perfuse the end organs and importantly maintain the vascular pressure head.

What is meant by vascular pressure head? Since there is more compliance in the venous system than in the arterial system, there exists a forward drive of blood from higher pressure to lower pressure, as illustrated in Fig. 13.8.

This pressure head is essential for the forward flow of blood and for sustaining the return of blood flow back to the heart from the venous system. Therefore, as cardiac output drops,

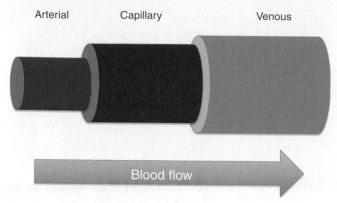

Arterial Capillary Venous

Blood flow

FIG. 13.8 The vascular pressure head as a mechanism for driving the forward flow of blood.

maintaining MAP with pressors through an increase in SVR only translates into an improvement in cardiac output from improvement in vascular pressure head leading to better venous return and ultimately better forward flow. If not, then increasing MAP with escalating pressors may only function to worsen overall perfusion.

Improvement in cardiac output with ECMO allows for a decrease in SVR needed to maintain this forward flow, improving blood flow to the end organs. Additionally, reducing the dose of pressors mitigates the adverse effects that high-dose pressors can have on cardiac output, such as worsening pulmonary vascular resistance/right ventricular afterload.

Effect #3: Perfuse Visceral Organs

Imagine the normal flow of blood out of the heart. It flows past the aortic valve into the ascending aorta and down the descending aorta. Within the next 12–18 inches it perfuses the liver, kidneys, intestines and mesentery, and entire abdomen. The lack of blood flow in cardiogenic shock causes a decline in blood flow to these essential organs as indicated by worsening lactate levels, liver enzymes, and renal function tests.

Now let's imagine what happens in ECMO. You have a column of oxygenated blood that is directed through this entire path. The result can be a rapid improvement in the perfusion of all of these organs (Fig. 13.9).

As perfusion is restored, you may witness a rapid improvement in urine output (minutes), lactate clearance/gut function (hours), and liver enzymes (days). The degree of this improvement is dependent on the extent that the injury was due to lack of perfusion rather than permanent damage. Patients with the latter fall into the "too far gone category" where ECMO may be of less benefit. However, teasing out where that line exists can be challenging when selecting patients for ECMO.

The result of these changes is a potential reversal of the vasodilatory effect of acidosis/renal failure/liver injury.

Effect #4: Provide Oxygen

Just as hypoxia exacerbates the vicious cycle, worsening delivery of oxygen to the coronary circulation, ECMO provides oxygen to the hypoxic patient in cardiogenic shock, mitigating this adverse effect. Oxygenated blood from the ECMO circuit can improve the overall delivery of oxygen which can translate to improved perfusion to multiple organ systems. However, this may be potentiated by the nature of the retrograde circulation.

$DO_2 \implies CO \times Hb \times SO_2$

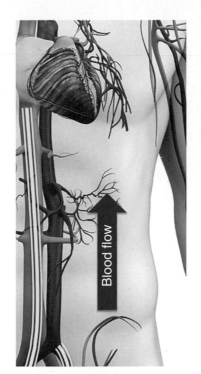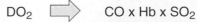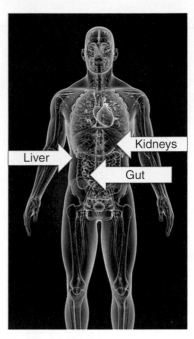

FIG. 13.9 The impact of ECMO blood flow on visceral organ perfusion. (From SciePro/Shutterstock.com and Sciencepics/Shutterstock.com.)

Effect #5: Support the Right Ventricle

By now you have likely developed a newfound respect for the role of the right ventricle in shock. While the left ventricle is responsible for the flow of blood to the rest of the body, it is completely dependent on the right ventricle, as the right ventricular cardiac output is the primary contributor to left ventricular preload. Thus the effects of right ventricular preload and afterload can impact the perfusion of the entire body.

Right ventricular afterload can be crushing. Causes of elevated pulmonary pressures include high left-sided pressures, hypoxia, poor pulmonary compliance, and hypercapnia. Improvement in oxygenation/CO_2 clearance from the ECMO circuit as well as improved acidosis from splanchnic perfusion can help to improve right ventricular afterload.

Additionally, in contrast to the effect of VV ECMO, the effect of VA ECMO on the right ventricle extends beyond afterload reduction. This is because any blood flow to the ECMO circuit represents blood that is drained from the right side, decompressing the right heart. If the right heart is over-distended to the point that it is impeding the filling of the left side of the heart, then this flow of blood will function to further improve overall perfusion (Fig. 13.10).

Effect # 6: Retrograde Blood Flow and the Left Ventricle

The flow of blood from the ECMO circuit exerts the opposite effect on the left ventricle in peripheral ECMO. While blood is drained away from the right ventricle in the venous circulation, it flows against the left ventricle since it is directed from the femoral artery up the aorta into the arterial circulation. Consequently, this flow and direction of blood *increases* left ventricular afterload and works against left ventricular cardiac output (Fig. 13.11).

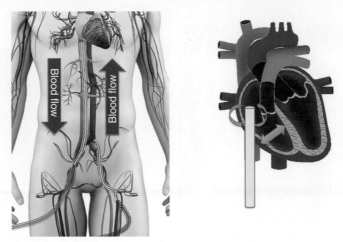

FIG. 13.10 VA ECMO as a mechanism of supporting the right ventricle. (From SciePro/Shutterstock.com and Ody_Stocker/Shutterstock.com.)

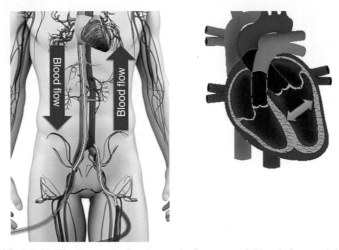

FIG. 13.11 The impact of retrograde flow on a failing left ventricle. (From SciePro/Shutterstock.com and Ody_Stocker/Shutterstock.com.)

Having an appreciation for the effects/limitations of this retrograde flow is a cornerstone of both the selection and management of VA ECMO. We will review the details of retrograde flow in detail in the next chapter.

PUTTING IT TOGETHER: VA ECMO AND THE VICIOUS CYCLE OF CARDIOGENIC SHOCK

In this chapter, we took a closer look at the vicious cycle of cardiogenic shock, getting a better sense of how the effects can spiral out of control. Rather than simply the consequence of low cardiac output, the cycle is the result of the compounding effects on multiple phenomena. The confluence of these effects is what dictates the rationale for VA ECMO, particularly, for which patients would be well suited. The higher the anticipated benefits and the lower the limitations will dictate the degree that VA ECMO will be of benefit to any individual patient. Let's review the effects that we discussed with attention to the effect ECMO will have:

✓	Decreased cardiac output
✓	Decreased coronary perfusion
⊘	Increased LV distension
✓	Hypoxia → coronary hypoxia
✓	Acidosis → vasodilation
✓	Acute kidney injury/fluid retention
✓	Worsening RV afterload
✓	Increased RV distension
✓	Pressors/fluid worsening RV

You will notice that VA ECMO has a positive effect on the majority of phenomena associated with cardiogenic shock, with the notable exception of increased left ventricular distension, which can potentially be worsened due to retrograde flow. Understanding retrograde flow is essential to understand the effect of deploying VA ECMO in this patient population, which is why we will dedicate the next chapter solely to the physiology of this phenomenon.

SUGGESTED READING

Beard, D. A., & Feigl, E. O. (2011). Understanding Guyton's venous return curves. *American Journal of Physiology-Heart and Circulatory Physiology., 301*(3), H629–H633.

Jones, T. L., Nakamura, K., & McCabe, J. M. (2019). Cardiogenic shock: evolving definitions and future directions in management. *Open Heart., 6*(1), e000960.

Werdan, K., Gielen, S., Ebelt, H., & Hochman, J. S. (2014). Mechanical circulatory support in cardiogenic shock. *European Heart Journal., 35*(3), 156–167.

14

Physiology of Retrograde Flow

There is nothing intuitive about retrograde flow.

You are pumping blood in one direction into the arterial system, which is the opposite direction that blood is supposed to flow. At first glance, this seems that it wouldn't make sense. Doesn't the aorta just become engorged? Does blood continue flowing backwards through the heart/lungs into the venous system? What happens to the tissues that are distal to the cannula (Fig. 14.1)?

Overall, retrograde flow involves understanding the overall directions of blood flow from the heart, the extracorporeal membrane oxygenation (ECMO) circuit, and throughout the vascular system. In this chapter, we will explore these as well as the potential effects that these can have on the body.

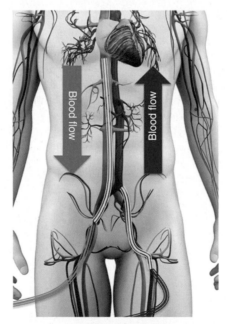

FIG. 14.1 Retrograde blood flow in VA ECMO. (Modified from SciePro/Shutterstock.com.)

THE DIRECTIONAL FLOW OF THE VASCULAR SYSTEM

If the network of blood vessels in the body was just a static system, then many of the above questions would hold true. However, as we have alluded to, the arterial/capillary/venous network functions as a very dynamic system that functions to drive blood flow forward, facilitating the forward/antegrade flow of blood.

How is this accomplished? The muscular arteries/arterioles contract along with the heart to drive blood forward, and the valved system of the veins accommodates this forward flow to eliminate pooling of blood, which may cause back pressure.

The overall effect is a high-pressure system that exists in the arterial circulation and a lower pressure system that exists in the venous system. This pressure differential drives blood forward and is responsible for filling pressure to the right side of the heart.

This vascular phenomenon is essential to answering our initial questions on blood flow during VA ECMO. What prevents blood from just engorging the aorta or continuing to flow backwards? How does any blood make it to the venous system where it can get drained by the venous cannula? The answer lies in this antegrade flow of the vascular system (Fig. 14.2).

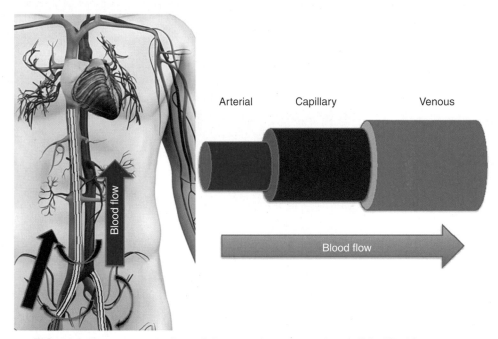

FIG. 14.2 The antegrade flow of the vascular pressure head. (Modified from SciePro/Shutterstock.com.)

Even if the heart is not beating at all (a phenomenon not uncommon in veno-arterial [VA] ECMO) there will still be antegrade flow from the arterial system through the capillary system into the venous system that allows for venous return. This antegrade flow of the vascular system can feasibly be driven by the ECMO flow, as the flow of blood from the ECMO circuit into the arterial circulation can serve to increase arterial pressure, increasing this pressure differential between arterial and venous systems.

THE NECESSITY OF RETROGRADE FLOW

Retrograde flow is a necessary consequence of peripherally inserted veno-arterial [VA] ECMO in adults. The intuitive manner of providing arterial blood flow would be antegrade, in order to pump blood in the direction of the heart and vascular system. However, there are both anatomic and functional limitations to doing so.

Accessing the heart/aorta directly requires surgical exposure. The carotid artery is used in children but is prohibitively risky in adults. The axillary artery can accommodate antegrade flow but is small enough that access requires grafting rather than percutaneous cannulation. This leaves us with the femoral artery, which is large enough to accommodate a cannula in most cases and can be accessed percutaneously, but requires flow to be directed retrograde through the aorta.

Let's now consider the physiologic effects of this retrograde flow.

The Effect of Retrograde Flow on the Left Ventricle

One of the most important implications of this retrograde flow is the effect on the left ventricle. The effect can be summarized in one word: afterload.

Remember afterload is the pressure that the heart must push against. You will remember from our initial introduction to afterload that the left heart is fairly tolerant of afterload, especially compared to the right heart (Fig. 14.3).

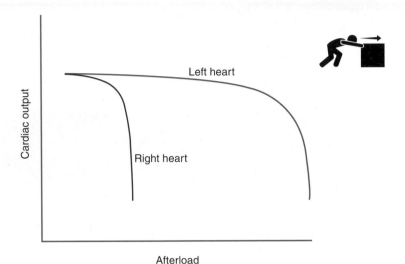

FIG. 14.3 Effects of afterload on the right and left heart. (Modified from Leremy/Stock Illustrations /Shutterstock.)

The primary reason for this tolerance is the function and anatomy of the left heart, which is more muscular and able to tolerate a higher pressure to work against. However, there is another phenomenon to consider, namely that as afterload increases, cardiac output drops. This in turn decreases mean arterial pressure (MAP), which decreases afterload.

In VA ECMO, this phenomenon is not necessarily the case, where the ECMO blood flow/afterload remains constant if the native cardiac output drops. This may mean that the effect of afterload due to retrograde flow will be more profound than would be normally observed if ECMO was not in place. The impact on the heart might be minimal or could lead to complete left ventricular dysfunction.

LEFT VENTRICULAR AFTERLOAD SENSITIVITY

Up until this point, we have generally described the afterload sensitivity of the left ventricle compared to the right ventricle, but there can also be a range of afterload sensitivity of the left ventricle depending on the clinical scenario. Let's consider the afterload effect of retrograde flow due to VA ECMO in two cases of cardiogenic shock.

Patient 1: Pulmonary embolism with preserved left ventricular function
Patient 2: Left anterior descending lesion with ischemic left ventricle

If both patients were placed on VA ECMO for cardiogenic shock, the responsiveness of their left ventricles may be very different. Patient 1 would be more tolerant to retrograde flow, with minimal impact on left ventricular output, while Patient 2 will experience a significant drop-off in left ventricular function/output (Fig. 14.4).

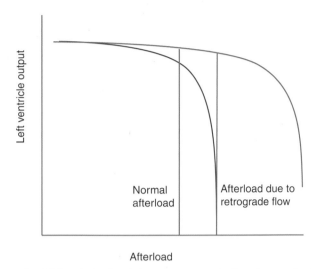

FIG. 14.4 The effect of additional afterload due to retrograde flow in a patient with primary right heart failure (green) versus primary left heart failure (red)

The degree of afterload sensitivity of the left ventricle will ultimately determine how it will be impacted by retrograde flow. In a case like Patient 1, there may be little to no effect of retrograde flow on the left ventricle, as the cardiogenic shock is only due to the failing right ventricle. In contrast, Patient 2 may experience a host of adverse effects to include worsening of the ischemia that caused the shock in the first place.

Let's further review these adverse effects of retrograde flow.

Adverse Effects of Retrograde Flow on the Left Ventricle

Imagine the case of Patient 2, our patient with ischemic cardiomyopathy and cardiogenic shock placed on VA ECMO. We gradually begin increasing the blood flow and notice a consequent increase in the MAP. But as MAP increases, you look at the arterial line tracing and notice a gradual narrowing, with a smaller and smaller difference in the pulse pressure. Continuing to increase the blood flow, the arterial line becomes flat. What is happening here?

As we have established to this point, the afterload has increased to the point that it has overwhelmed the ability of the left ventricle to eject blood. It may be still contracting (barely) but these movements may be insufficient to overcome the afterload from the ECMO circuit and the aortic valve may not actually open.

Thrombosis

If the aortic valve is not opening or is barely opening, this increases the static blood that exists around the valve and in the left ventricle. Even if anticoagulation is administered, the risk of clot formation is increased, a dangerous possibility in the arterial circulation due to the risk of valvular damage, stroke, or embolization.

Increased Left Ventricular Distension

As pulse pressure decreases and less blood is ejected out of the left ventricle, the ventricle can continue filling and become dilated.

How Do You Get Left Ventricular Distension If You Are on Complete ECMO Support?

If ECMO is draining all of the blood from the right ventricle and returning it to the arterial circulation, shouldn't there be no blood that is returning to the left ventricle? Unfortunately, this is not the case, even if the ECMO circuit is completely bypassing the heart. This is because there are blood vessels that drain directly into the left side of the heart as part of a normal, anatomic shunt. The cardiac veins drain into the Thebesian veins, some of which drain into the left side of the heart. Additionally, the bronchial circulation arises from the aorta, giving rise to the bronchial veins which drain directly into the left atrium. This means that even if your ECMO flow is greater than the cardiac output, the left ventricle will start to distend.

Increased Wall Stress on the Myocardium

Now you have a distended heart and increased afterload, both of which increase the amount of tension on the muscular ventricular wall. This increased wall tension decreases blood supply by compressing on the blood vessels supplying the myocardial cells of the heart. This can lead to worsening ischemia and myocardial damage, which can further any ischemia that precipitated the initial injury.

Elevated Pulmonary Pressures and Pulmonary Edema

As left ventricular pressures increase, it leads to increasing pressure in the left atrium, which eventually translates to increasing pressure in the pulmonary venous circulation. The result is higher hydrostatic pressure and accumulation of edema into the lungs. Pulmonary edema increases pulmonary shunt and will result in worsening oxygenation of any blood that is coming from the right side of the heart through the lungs. The effects of this hypoxic blood can be profound as we will discuss later (Fig. 14.5).

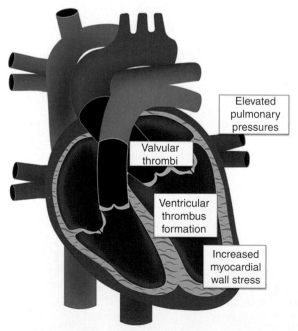

FIG. 14.5 Adverse effects of retrograde flow. (Modified from Ody_Stocker/Shutterstock.com.)

Venting the Left Ventricle

Because of the damaging effects of left ventricular distension, there exists a rationale for venting the left ventricle. This is an ability to allow blood to flow out of the left ventricle, improving distension, and preventing/mitigating the negative effects detailed earlier. Venting is not universal and varies based on practice patterns. Some pathology (for example, pulmonary embolism/primary right ventricular failure with preserved left ventricular function) may not need to be vented. However, once adverse effects of left ventricular distension such as thrombosis or pulmonary edema accumulate, it can be more difficult to manage, and the risk exists for rapid decompensation.

Potential options for venting include the following:

- **Chemical vent:** Use of inotropes to improve contractility and facilitate ejection of blood from the left ventricle.
- **Intra-aortic balloon pump:** Pump placed into the aorta via the femoral artery, facilitating the forward flow of blood through a counterpulsating balloon. Decreases afterload and improves coronary perfusion.
- **Percutaneous left ventricular assist device:** Motorized device that can facilitate the flow of blood from the left ventricle to the aorta distal to the aortic valve. Can be placed percutaneously from the contralateral femoral artery or surgically from the axillary artery.
- **Surgical drain:** Drainage of blood directly from the left ventricle, usually in the form of a drain from the apex of the left ventricle that is connected to the drain side of the circuit (see Fig. 14.6A). Usually, this is much more common in central cannulation as placement of this drain requires surgical access.
- **PA drain:** Rarely, if unable to drain from any other source, drainage of blood from the pulmonary artery can decompress the left side of the heart by draining out blood from the pulmonary circulation (see Fig. 14.6B). Cardiogenic shock in the setting of mitral stenosis may require this strategy, for example.

Left ventricular vents such as inotropes, intra-aortic balloon pumps, and percutaneous left ventricular assist devices have the advantage of being a bridge that ECMO can be weaned to as native recovery continues to progress.

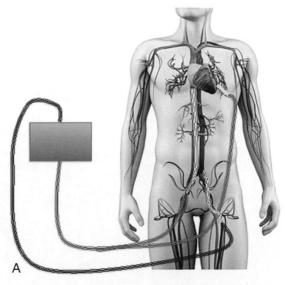

FIG. 14.6A Venting strategy: apical vent. (Modified from SciePro/Shutterstock.com.)

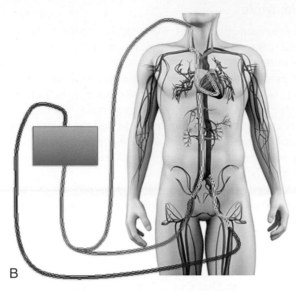

B

FIG. 14.6B Venting strategy: pulmonary artery (PA) drain. (Modified from SciePro/Shutterstock.com.)

WHICH WAY IS BLOOD FLOWING AGAIN?

One reason peripheral VA ECMO is confusing is we have to familiarize ourselves with competing directions of blood flow. We are accustomed to thinking of blood flow in one direction – out of the right heart, into the pulmonary circulation, into the left heart, out into the arterial circulation, across the vascular pressure head into the venous circulation, and into the right heart.

Now we have identified multiple competing directions of blood flow. Let's review in Fig. 14.7.

In the case of ECMO, we have drainage of venous blood into the ECMO circuit and return of oxygenated blood in a retrograde fashion as well as the maintenance of the vascular pressure head allowing for return of blood to the venous system and continued drainage through the circuit. We

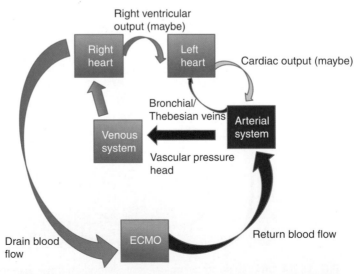

FIG. 14.7 Schematic of blood flow circulations on VA ECMO

also have drainage of bronchial/Thebesian veins into the left side of the heart. These circulations are maintained even if we are on complete ECMO support, with the heart doing nothing. On top of this, we can have antegrade blood flow from the right/left heart that can compete against the ECMO blood flow in the case of partial ECMO support or as the heart begins to recover. Let's now look at what this looks like clinically.

Competing Circulation on VA ECMO: Retrograde Versus Antegrade Blood Flow

The interplay between retrograde blood flow from the ECMO circuit and antegrade blood flow from the native heart/lungs is the fundamental dynamic to understand in peripheral VA ECMO. Understanding, identifying, and assessing these competing circulations will be essential to managing VA ECMO.

Let's return to our thought experiment, considering the physiology of our patient with ischemic cardiomyopathy. When we last left him, our flow was increased to the degree that there was no pulsatility on the arterial line, and the aortic valve was barely opening. (Fig. 14.8). Illustrates of what this would look like for the rest of the body.

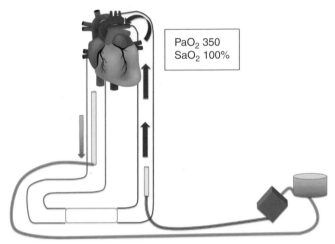

FIG. 14.8 VA ECMO oxygenation in patient with minimal native cardiac output. (Modified from Ody_Stocker/Shutterstock.com.)

As you can see, since there is no forward/antegrade flow from the heart, the oxygen content of blood returning from the ECMO circuit is exactly what the body sees. This includes the arterial circulation from the aorta all the way up to the coronary ostia. The oxygen delivery of the circuit translates so directly to the oxygen delivery of the body that we may consider decreasing FiO_2 to the ECMO circuit, so as not to cause cerebral damage from hyperoxia.

In this case, you have complete and efficient delivery of oxygen and all of the benefits of VA ECMO discussed in Chapter 13 (perfusion of abdominal organs, support of right heart, support of MAP, etc.). However, these benefits have to be weighed against the harmful effects of left ventricular distension/stasis.

You go home for the night, and return the next morning. To your pleasant surprise, you note that there is now pulsatility on the arterial line. An echocardiogram later in the morning shows an improvement in the left ventricular function with opening of the aortic valve. However, when you review the labs for the morning, you note that there is a PaO_2 of 60 mmHg on the blood gas where this had been 350 mmHg yesterday. What happened? Why did the oxygenation of the blood decrease?

In this case, we are seeing evidence of competing circulations (Fig. 14.9). While you had one circulation from the ECMO circuit that was unencumbered yesterday, today, there is clearly evidence that these two circulations are competing against each other. There is still blood draining from the arterial to the venous system via the vascular pressure head, however this is done via two competing flows, much like two hoses aimed into a drain will still drain in the same direction.

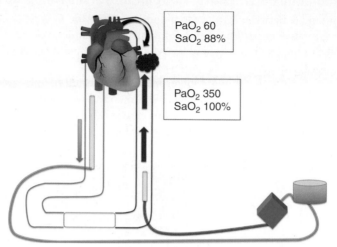

PaO$_2$ 60
SaO$_2$ 88%

PaO$_2$ 350
SaO$_2$ 100%

FIG. 14.9 VA ECMO oxygenation in patient with improving cardiac function. (Modified from Ody_Stocker/Shutterstock.com.)

How can we assess these two flows? Which blood flow is supplying what organ? Can we quantify this?

In general, ECMO blood flow should be assessed in the context of how perfusion is maintained. In other words, ECMO blood flow should be titrated based on the clinical indicators of perfusion: assessing whether we are maintaining an adequate MAP and urine output, reducing pressors, with lactate and liver function tests normalizing. If we are not maintaining these endpoints, then we need to address ECMO blood flow or adjust other support.

However, as competing antegrade flow from the heart/lungs increases, we will need to understand and quantify the effect of this circulation. We will do this by assessing the effect of this competing circulation on oxygenation.

Assessing Oxygenation of the Native Circulation: Role of the Right Radial Arterial Line

We now see that we have evidence of a mixing cloud somewhere between the heart and the ECMO return cannula, where blood proximal to the mixing cloud reflects the oxygenation of the native heart/lungs while blood distal to the mixing cloud reflects the oxygenation of the ECMO circuit.

Often teams will opt to place a right radial arterial line in patients with VA ECMO. Why is this? Looking at Fig. 14.10, as blood travels out of the heart, past the aortic valve, the first vessels supplied are the coronary arteries, the innominate artery, which gives rise to the right internal carotid artery, and the left internal carotid artery. Usually, this works in the body's favor having the coronary and cerebral blood vessels supplied first, prioritizing the oxygenation of these organ systems (Fig. 14.10).

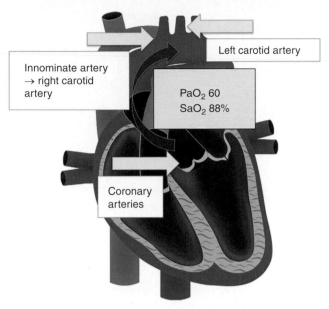

FIG. 14.10 Blood vessels initially supplied from blood leaving the left ventricle. (Modified from Ody_Stocker/Shutterstock.com.)

However, when we are on ECMO, and experiencing recovering cardiac function, this blood will reflect the oxygenation of whatever the lungs are able to supply (the saturation being 88% in Fig. 14.10).

The value of a right radial arterial line is that it reflects the oxygenation of what is being supplied to the innominate artery and will give the best sense of the circulation that is coming from the heart/lungs since it is the most proximal sample of the aortic supply that can be taken. If blood is oxygenated to the right radial artery, the assumption is that the same or greater oxygenated blood is being supplied to the cerebral circulation.

WORSENING HYPOXIA WHILE ON VA ECMO: IDENTIFICATION AND MITIGATION

Let's return to our patient. It is now ECMO day 3. The heart has been slowly recovering over the last several days. The chest X-ray has been gradually worsening, likely from an aspiration pneumonia that occurred during the initial arrest that triggered the cardiogenic shock.

We have been following blood gas results from a femoral line that was left in the contralateral groin as well as from a right radial arterial line that was placed and have noticed a gradual worsening of the oxygenation of the blood from the arterial line. The most recent blood gas results are as follows:

Right radial line ABG: 7.35, $PaCO_2$ 52, **PaO_2 60, SaO_2 75%**
Femoral line ABG: 7.49, $PaCO_2$ 30, **PaO_2 350, SaO_2 100%**

What explains the different results? As you can deduce, the femoral arterial line is reflecting the circulation from the ECMO circuit while the radial arterial line is reflecting the circulation from the heart and lungs.

This can be a common phenomenon to monitor on VA ECMO – upper body hypoxemia combined with lower body hyperoxia, sometimes referred to as harlequin phenomenon. The two components of this phenomenon are improving cardiac function and worsening pulmonary function (Fig. 14.11).

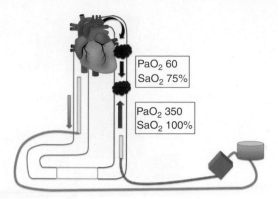

FIG. 14.11 VA ECMO oxygenation in patient with improving cardiac function and worsening lung function. (Modified from Ody_Stocker/Shutterstock.com.)

Why is this phenomenon common? It is a common pattern to see a drop in native cardiac output initially, in the initial phases of the injury, due to the effect of the afterload from the retrograde flow of the ECMO circuit, which can then slowly improve over the course of the next several days. However, it is also a common pattern to see the worsening of pulmonary function over the course of several days, either due to pneumonia as in this case or pulmonary edema due to insufficient left ventricular venting/volume overload/etc.

As a consequence, we must always maintain vigilance in monitoring for this phenomenon. If arterial blood gases are checked from a femoral arterial line, or even from a left-sided radial arterial line, the possibility exists of being falsely reassured of adequate oxygenation to the cerebral and coronary blood vessels, by sampling blood that is reflective of the ECMO circulation rather than the native heart/lungs. By checking for adequate oxygenation of the blood coming from the native heart/lungs, we are ensuring that oxygenated blood is being delivered to the coronary and cerebral vessels so as not to worsen any injury.

The second step is mitigation and correction of hypoxia once the phenomenon is recognized. If you recognize hypoxia in blood to the right radial arterial line, then we must improve oxygenation by optimizing the native heart and lungs. This can be done in a variety of ways to include:

- **Increase support from the ventilator**. Increasing PEEP or FiO_2 will usually improve oxygenation of blood being ejected from the native heart/lungs. Remember that this approach is counterproductive if you have to escalate support to the degree that it is injurious to the native heart/lungs.
- **Diurese/treat underlying cause**. If the cause is due to pulmonary edema, diuresis can help to fix the underlying pulmonary issues and will prevent from having to escalate support from the ventilator, as noted earlier. If due to other pulmonary etiologies (pneumonia, mucous plugging, bronchospasm) then attentive management of the underlying cause (timely antibiotics, secretion clearance, administration of bronchodilators) can be of benefit.
- **Address left ventricular venting strategy**. Intermittently, this hypoxia can be due to insufficient venting strategy. Mitigating strategies can include adding inotropes, adding another form of mechanical circulatory support (balloon pump, percutaneous left ventricular support device, etc.), or escalating to a more robust form of support (such as a surgically implanted temporary ventricular support device).
- **Transition ECMO configuration to Veno-arterial venous (VAV) ECMO**. If all else fails, and upper body hypoxia is refractory to any other interventions, then a transition to VAV

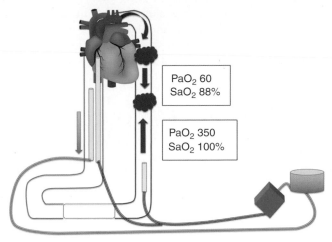

FIG. 14.12 VA ECMO oxygenation in patient on VAV ECMO. (Modified from Ody_Stocker/Shutterstock.com.)

ECMO may allow for circulatory support, while also providing oxygenated blood to the venous side of the circulation and improving hypoxia (illustrated in Fig. 14.12). Let's examine this support configuration in a little more detail.

VAV ECMO in Supporting Upper Body Hypoxemia in Setting of Cardiogenic Shock

When we use VAV ECMO in this setting, we are adding a venous cannula either in the femoral vein or in the internal jugular/subclavian vein and connecting it to the return line of the ECMO circuit via a plastic Y connector (Fig. 14.13).

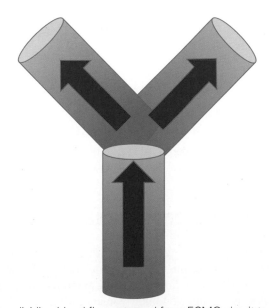

FIG. 14.13 Y connector dividing blood flow returned from ECMO circuit to two different cannulas

This connection divides oxygenated blood returning from the ECMO membrane/pump between the venous return cannula and the arterial cannula. Doing so allows for cardiac support and respiratory support simultaneously. The more blood flow that is directed toward the arterial cannula, the greater the cardiac support, while the more blood flow directed toward the venous return cannula, the greater the respiratory support.

TITRATION OF SUPPORT ON VAV ECMO

Let's say you transition our patient to VAV ECMO, in order to allow for better oxygenation. You cut in the Y connection and go back on flow. How would you imagine that flow is being divided between the arterial and venous limbs?

As you might have figured, based on our discussion of flow dynamics, the venous limb will have a lower resistance and, therefore, all else being equal, blood would flow preferentially into the venous limb (Fig. 14.14).

Therefore, on initiation of VAV ECMO, excess resistance will have to be placed on the venous limb, whether in the form of a partially occlusive pump clamp or an adjustable clamp. After this, then flow can be adjusted based on the desired support to the venous or the arterial side.

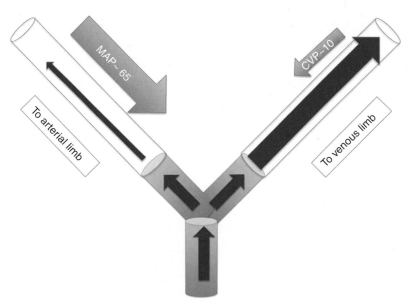

FIG. 14.14 Preferential flow of blood toward venous limb on VAV ECMO CVP, Central venous pressure; MAP, mean arterial pressure.

HOW DO YOU KNOW HOW BLOOD IS BEING DIVIDED?

After going on VAV ECMO, you can attach a flow probe to the arterial limb. This will measure how much blood is going into the arterial side of the circulation (say 2 L/min). This can be subtracted from the total blood flow to give the amount of blood going to the venous cannula. So, if total blood flow is 5 L/min, you know you are giving 2 L/min to the arterial limb and 3 L/min to the venous limb.

If you want to then increase the arterial blood flow to achieve 2.5 L/min of flow, you can attempt to tighten the clamp on the venous limb, increasing the resistance, and directing more blood to the arterial side. However, at a certain point, you may reach diminishing returns, as tightening the occlusion to the venous limb may increase the overall resistance applied to the circuit and decrease the overall blood flow.

PUTTING IT ALL TOGETHER

Understanding retrograde physiology is essential to understanding peripherally inserted VA ECMO support. Knowing the impact of flow of this nature and being able to identify and predict the risks associated with this flow is what defines candidacy for VA ECMO as opposed to other forms of mechanical circulatory support. The degree that a patient with cardiac failure will be able to tolerate this retrograde flow is the fundamental component of whether or not they should be supported with VA ECMO.

This dynamic changes slightly when we think of the physiology of centrally cannulated ECMO, which is what we will focus on in the next chapter.

SUGGESTED READING

Avalli, L., Maggioni, E., Sangalli, F., Favini, G., Formica, F., Fumagalli, R. et al. (2011). Percutaneous left-heart decompression during extracorporeal membrane oxygenation: an alternative to surgical and transseptal venting in adult patients. *Asaio Journal, 57*(1), 38–40.

Baldetti, L., Gramegna, M., Beneduce, A., Melillo, F., Moroni, F., Calvo, F., et al. (2020). Strategies of left ventricular unloading during VA-ECMO support: a network meta-analysis.. *International Journal of Cardiology, 312*, 16–21.

Funk, D. J., Jacobsohn, E., & Kumar, A. (2013). The role of venous return in critical illness and shock—part I: physiology. *Critical Care Medicine, 41*(1), 255–262.

Fux, T., Holm, M., Corbascio, M., van der Linden, J., Lund, L. H. et al. (2017). Pre-implant outcome predictors in patients with refractory cardiogenic shock supported with VA-ECMO. Journal of the American College of Cardiology, 70(16), 2094–2096.

Tarazi, R. C., & Levy, M. N. (1982). Cardiac responses to increased afterload. State-of-the-art review. *Hypertension, 4*(3_pt_2), 8–18.

Zweck, E., Thayer, K. L., Helgestad, O. K. L., Kanwar, M., Ayouty, M., Garan, A. R., et al. (2021). Phenotyping cardiogenic shock. Journal of the American Heart Association, 10(14), e020085.

15

Central Veno-Arterial ECMO Physiology

We will now continue our exploration of VA ECMO physiology by considering the physiology of centrally cannulated VA ECMO. The proportion of central cannulation is largely facility dependent. While some programs mainly rely on peripherally placed ECMO cannulas, others have a significant percentage of central cannulation. Regardless, it is important to understand the physiologic subtleties unique to this configuration.

PRIMARY CENTRAL CANNULATION CONFIGURATION

As we learned in our configurations discussion in Chapter 8, central cannulation involves cannulation directly to the heart and great vessels. The usual configuration is a dual-stage cannula implanted directly to the right atrium with a cannula implanted directly onto the aorta with an additional vent of the left ventricle either by a drain of the pulmonary veins or directly from the left ventricular apex (Fig. 15.1).

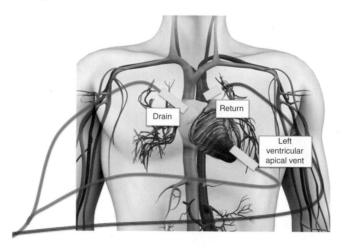

FIG. 15.1 Central cannulation configuration. (Modified from SciePro/Shutterstock.com.)

ANTEGRADE FLOW AND PERFUSION OF CORONARY ARTERIES

The result is the ability to provide antegrade flow that bypasses both the heart and lungs. The physiologic advantages over retrograde support should be immediately apparent. Retrograde flow is no longer required, meaning that everything that is flowing from the extracorporeal membrane oxygenation (ECMO) circuit is what the body is receiving. The adverse effects of retrograde flow that we discussed in Chapter 14 (left ventricular afterload, competing flows, upper body hypoxia, etc.) are significantly mitigated in this configuration. Specifically, perfusion of the cerebral vessels is much more reliable, as the aortic cannula will be providing antegrade flow prior to the takeoff of the innominate and left common carotid artery (Fig. 15.2).

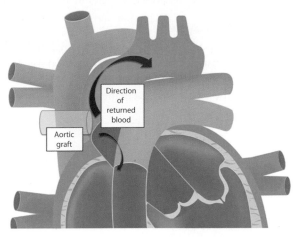

FIG. 15.2 Antegrade and retrograde blood flow from aortic graft. (Modified from Ody_Stocker/Shutterstock.com.)

Perfusion of the coronary arteries on the other hand is more dependent on retrograde flow from the cannula. While the majority of flow is directed in an antegrade direction, there is a small proportion of blood that flows back towards the heart which is needed for provision of oxygenated blood to the coronary arteries supplying the heart.

The second major advantage of this form of support is the amount of flow that can be provided. Remember that in peripherally inserted VA ECMO, we have a distinct limitation of flow that exists due to the retrograde nature of support. We can increase retrograde blood flow, but at a certain point, the advantages of higher ECMO blood flow (better perfusion/support) are outweighed by the disadvantages of retrograde support (left ventricular afterload, aortic valve closure, pulmonary edema).

The limits of retrograde flow to the overall amount of flow provided do not exist in central cannulation; therefore, central cannulation can be an option for a higher degree of support that can be considered on initiation of ECMO or as an upgrade of support. While retrograde limits to flow do not exist, limits to flow on central cannulation do exist.

LIMITS TO BLOOD FLOW ON CENTRAL CANNULATION

Let's envision a patient on central cannulation. As we review the clinical data, we note that the lactate is rising slightly, urine output is dropping off, mean arterial pressure is low, and venous oxygen saturation is low. We conclude that we are not supporting her optimally and want to increase our ECMO blood flow. What are the limits to flow in this patient?

Flow Limit #1: Limit of the ECMO Circuit/Pump

All of the considerations for flow limitation that we considered in Chapter 10 still apply. There is still a maximal flow that the oxygenator can accommodate as well as the preload dependence/afterload sensitivity of the pump.

Preload dependence can still be a major limit to flow. Even though the cannula is placed directly into the right atrium and the collapsibility of the inferior vena cava (IVC) is not a limit to flow, a lack of venous return in the form of hypovolemia/bleeding can represent a major limit to flow.

Flow Limit #2: Mean Arterial Pressure

Afterload to the pump includes anything post pump to include tubing, oxygenator, cannulas, and ultimately mean arterial pressure. As flow increases, this can increase mean arterial pressure and increase the pressure differential that the pump will have to overcome. As this pressure differential increases, the pump may have to run at a higher rate of revolutions per minute (RPMs), which increases the risk of hemolysis.

Flow Limit #3: Pressures of the System

As flows across the pump increase, the post-pump pressure will increase as well. Higher pressures are sensed across the entire post-pump circuit, from the oxygenator all the way down to the cannula. The difference in pressure differential at normal (Fig. 15.3) and higher blood flows is illustrated in Fig. 15.4. The higher the blood flow, the higher the post-pump pressures will be (points 2 and 3).

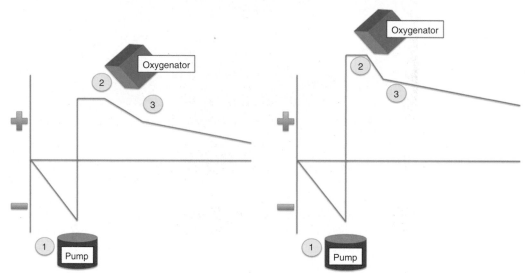

FIG. 15.3 and 15.4 Pressure differentials at normal blood flow and higher blood flow in central VA ECMO

The pressure limits of the system can be usually defined and set by individual facilities. The higher these pressures, the higher the risk of damage to the oxygenator, graft, or blood vessels into which the cannula is implanted.

Flow Limit #4: Overflow of the System

At a certain point, blood can overflow the arterial system, causing damage to blood vessels or end organs. In general, as with any type of support, excessive flow should be minimized. Rather, the focus should remain on maintaining the lowest possible blood flow that can achieve the desired physiologic endpoints.

LEFT VENTRICULAR VENTING IN CENTRAL CANNULATION

Just as with peripheral cannulation, venting of the left side of the heart should warrant careful consideration. Without venting, adverse effects of left ventricular distension can occur, to include pulmonary edema, left ventricular stasis, thrombosis, and increased wall stress/worsening of myocardial ischemia.

How Does Left Ventricular Distension Happen in Central Cannulation?

Left ventricular distension in central ECMO may not be immediately intuitive. The blood is antegrade, and higher flows can allow for complete bypass of the pulmonary circulation. However, even if the blood flow of the ECMO circuit is high enough that there is no blood leaving the right ventricle into the pulmonary artery, there is blood that still drains into the heart. As we previously mentioned, the blood supply of the bronchial circulation comes off the aorta and drains directly into the pulmonary veins, which return blood to the left heart. In a similar way, some of the small cardiac endocardial veins, referred to as the Thebesian vein, drain blood directly into the left ventricle rather than into the coronary sinus.

It is these venous blood vessels that can contribute to ongoing left ventricular distension even if the heart is completely bypassed.

The left ventricle drain, whether it is from the pulmonary vein or the left ventricular apex, can be connected to the drainage side of the circuit, via Y connector. Even though it is "red" oxygenated blood, it is used as a drain as the negative pressure is needed to pull the blood. The drain should be connected to a clamp and flow probe, in order to regulate the amount of blood being drained. Enough blood should be drained from the left side of the heart to minimize the effects of left ventricular distension while simultaneously allowing for enough cardiac filling to allow for ejection. Regulating this will require careful examination for pulmonary edema as well as echocardiographic findings (to ensure sufficient draining) while also observing for pulsatility (to ensure sufficient filling).

REGULATION OF BLOOD FLOW ON CENTRAL VA ECMO

We discussed the limits to blood flow earlier. However, how much blood flow should be targeted; the maximum possible or some other target? The answer lies in the goals of support in the clinical situation.

The clinical spectrum may look something like the illustration in Fig. 15.5. Initially, the goal is just trying to maintain perfusion targets, then allowing for cardiac rest/buying time to wait for further takebacks/surgeries, and finally ending with cardiac recovery and ability to wean. Cardiac rest is the concept of giving the heart time to recover after its injury without worsening myocardial damage due to excessive filling or escalating doses of inotropes. The lower the blood flow, the more cardiac filling that we allow, with the aim of allowing for some contribution of the native heart and lungs.

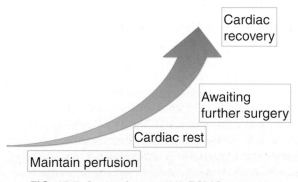

FIG. 15.5 Goals of central VA ECMO support

The other reason to allow for some cardiac activity is to allow for flow across the pulmonary vascular bed. As the ECMO blood flow increases and the amount of blood leaving the right heart continues to decrease, there is progressive stasis of blood in the pulmonary arteries/veins. This will increase the risk of thrombosis even in the presence of anticoagulation.

REGULATION OF SWEEP GAS FLOW ON CENTRAL VA ECMO

The physiology of central antegrade flow requires more careful attention and regulation of the post-oxygenator blood. Normally, the post-oxygenator blood gas is used to evaluate the health of the *membrane* oxygenator, relying on the patient arterial blood gas to determine the effect of what is going on with the patient, after the mixing of native and ECMO circulation.

In central cannulation, the blood returning from the oxygenator will closely resemble what is leaving the oxygenator. This means that if the post-oxygenator PaO_2 is 350 mmHg, then we can likely anticipate that the blood gas results from the arterial line will also have a PaO_2 close to 350 mmHg, especially if ECMO blood flow is the primary contributor to overall circulation (Fig. 15.6).

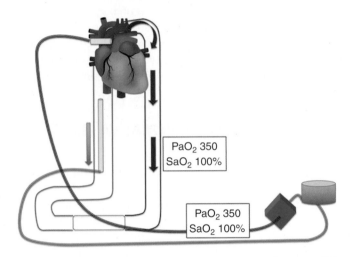

PaO$_2$ 350
SaO$_2$ 100%

PaO$_2$ 350
SaO$_2$ 100%

FIG. 15.6 Central cannulation and oxygen content of returned blood. (Modified from Ody_Stocker/Shutterstock.com.)

Why is this relevant? More oxygen is better, right?

Remember that optimal oxygen delivery requires well-saturated hemoglobin, with additional dissolved oxygen (PaO_2) contributing little to oxygen delivery. Excessive PaO_2 concentration, referred to as hyperoxia, does little to improve oxygen delivery to the peripheral tissue and can be harmful to the end organs, especially to the brain. This can be particularly relevant in the case of any brain that had any anoxic insult, such as in cardiac arrest, protracted hypoxia, or prolonged cardiopulmonary bypass run, all common in patients on central VA ECMO.

Also pay careful attention to CO_2 levels, adjusting sweep gas flow down as appropriate. In the same way that PaO_2 can easily be supraphysiologic in post-oxygenator blood, the efficiency of the membrane oxygenator in clearing CO_2 can lead to low levels of $PaCO_2$ in the post-oxygenator blood. Normally this does not matter as this blood mixes with CO_2 from the native circulation, giving a normalized CO_2 that can be adjusted with sweep gas flow. However, since there may be little to no mixing with native circulation in central VA ECMO, there is the possibility of hypocapnea in the arterial blood. Low arterial blood CO_2 levels can lead to further brain injury, by causing the constriction of cerebral blood vessels and decreasing the cerebral perfusion.

Therefore, pay close attention to the post-oxygenator/patient arterial blood gases, aiming for normal levels of $PaO_2/PaCO_2$. Often, close regulation of oxygenation of the post-oxygenator blood needs to be made – this may be time to use the FiO_2 dial on the oxygen blender, dialing back the FiO_2 to aim for normal PaO_2.

EFFECT OF NATIVE CARDIAC OUTPUT ON ANTEGRADE CENTRAL FLOW

The aforementioned phenomenon details the effects of central VA ECMO when the ECMO blood flow accounts for the majority of perfusion. However, as the heart recovers, there begins to be an effect of the native cardiac output. Let's explore how this manifests physiologically.

Let's say you are managing a patient on day 3 of his ECMO run. He was centrally cannulated for ECMO due to post-cardiotomy shock with a right atrial drain, an aortic return cannula, and a left ventricular apical vent. When you do your initial assessment, you note that the oxygen saturation is 88%.

HYPOXIA ON CENTRAL VA ECMO?

Although not as common as in peripheral VA ECMO, this can occur as the heart starts to recover and account for a greater percentage of overall perfusion. In this case, the blood flow from the heart/lungs is not competing against the blood flow from the ECMO circuit as with peripheral VA ECMO, but rather running in series with the ECMO circuit, like in VV ECMO (Fig. 15.7).

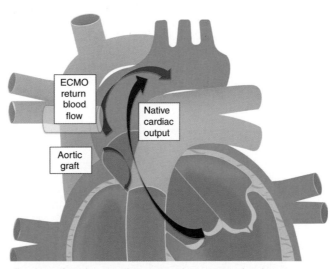

FIG. 15.7 Contribution of native cardiac output in a recovering heart on central VA ECMO. (Modified from Ody_Stocker/Shutterstock.com.)

The result is that much like VV ECMO, the ECMO circuit is only accounting for a proportion of the cardiac output. As the heart continues to recover, the saturation will more closely resemble the saturation of the blood returning to the left atrium from the pulmonary veins.

Although the oxygenation may not be optimal, this may represent a recovery of the cardiac function to such a degree that assessment for weaning may be possible.

PUTTING IT TOGETHER: THE RISKS/BENEFITS OF CENTRAL ECMO

To this point, central VA ECMO may seem like an attractive option. It is able to provide oxygenation, pulmonary, and cardiac support, without the strain on the right heart or left heart seen in VV ECMO or VA ECMO, respectively.

However, this does not mean that central ECMO is not without its disadvantages. The primary disadvantage involves the invasiveness of this configuration, often requiring sternotomy, access to heart/major blood vessels, and maintenance of an open chest. Complications can include bleeding, infection, stroke, need for subsequent operations, and heavy sedation/analgesia requirements. Additionally, maintaining an open chest can significantly limit mobility.

The benefits of antegrade flow should be weighed against these drawbacks/risks, when considering the configuration to support.

SUGGESTED READING

Cevasco, M., Takayama, H., Ando, M., Garan, A. R., Naka, Y., & Takeda, K., et al. (2019). Left ventricular distension and venting strategies for patients on venoarterial extracorporeal membrane oxygenation. *Journal of Thoracic Disease*, *11*(4), 1676.

Donker, D. W., Brodie, D., Henriques, J. P. S., & Broomé, M. (2019). Left ventricular unloading during veno-arterial ECMO: a review of percutaneous and surgical unloading interventions. *Perfusion*, *34*(2), 98–105.

Gu, K., Zhang, Y., Gao, B., Chang, Y., & Zeng, Y. (2016). Hemodynamic differences between central ECMO and peripheral ECMO: a primary CFD study. *Medical Science Monitor: International Medical Journal of Experimental and Clinical Research*, *22*, 717.

Lorusso, R., Raffa, G. M., Alenizy, K., Sluijpers, N., Makhoul, M., & Brodie, D., et al. (2019). Structured review of post-cardiotomy extracorporeal membrane oxygenation: part 1—adult patients. *The Journal of Heart and Lung Transplantation*, *38*(11), 1125–1143.

Raffa, G. M., Kowalewski, M., Brodie, D., Ogino, M., Whitman, G., & Meani, P., et al. (2019). Meta-analysis of peripheral or central extracorporeal membrane oxygenation in postcardiotomy and non-postcardiotomy shock. *The Annals of Thoracic Surgery*, *107*(1), 311–321.

PART IV

ECMO Management

16

Introduction to ECMO Management Principles

Hopefully by this point, you are starting to develop a much better sense of the principles at play when someone is on extracorporeal membrane oxygenation (ECMO). We started with the fundamentals, reviewing how oxygen is delivered throughout the body, how that system can break down, and the interventions to improve this delivery of oxygen, understanding that they can have dose-related toxicity that can compound with worsening respiratory/cardiac failure. We then introduced ECMO as a strategy that can mitigate that toxicity and were introduced to the components and configurations that we might come across. Finally, we explored the physiology of the various types of support, understanding the dynamics of flow, the capabilities of the membrane, and the rationale/limits of the various types of support.

This final section will now put attempt to put it all together, exploring the subtleties related to managing a patient on ECMO. The principles developed over the previous chapters will be fundamental, as they will form the foundation on which these management concepts are built.

THE CORNERSTONE OF ECMO MANAGEMENT: LESSEN TOXICITY

Let's return to our proposition that we are considering when it comes to the overall rationale of ECMO – namely that there are risks associated with ECMO; however, these risks can pay off in the long run if they mitigate the toxicity associated with conventional care (Fig. 16.1).

This proposition becomes the backbone of management when it comes to ECMO. Namely, ECMO only becomes advantageous to the degree that it mitigates the toxicity of support from conventional care.

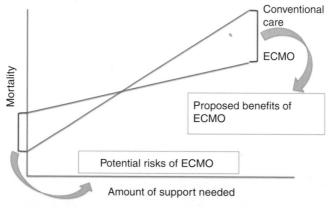

FIG. 16.1 Comparing the relative benefits/risks of ECMO v. conventional care

What Is Meant by Toxicity of Conventional Care?

Let's imagine a patient with no medical issues in the ICU with viral pneumonia and a superimposed bacterial pneumonia. He is intubated due to refractory hypoxia and is now on day 7 of his ICU course. The ventilator is clearly helping normalize his oxygen/CO_2 levels.

We often formulate our plan for how he will be managed by systems, from head to toe. Let's now go head to toe and speculate on the potential damaging effects related to ICU support that he is at risk for that has nothing to do with his inciting injury.

Neurologic: He is likely on sedation to facilitate synchrony with the ventilator, which is making him more delirious. He may be developing post traumatic stress disorder that can be related to oversedation or undersedation. He is likely having sleep-wake disturbances. He may be on paralytics due to hypoxia, which is increasing his risk of weakness.

Pulmonary: The ventilator may be damaging his alveoli causing excessive stretch and barotrauma/volutrauma. Even at low, "lung-protective" ventilator settings, there may be some alveoli that are overfilled (leading to barotrauma/volutrauma), while some are underfilled (leading to atelectotrauma).

Cardiac: Positive end-expiratory pressure (PEEP) from the ventilator may impair his ventricular filling. Pressors may be worsening his ability to adequately deliver oxygen and worsen ischemia to end organs. The ventilator may be worsening his right ventricle.

GI: Medications and immobility may decrease his gastric motility. Tube feeds may be inadequate to meet his caloric demands. The ventilator and steroids administered may lead to stress ulcers.

Renal: Pressors and excessive volume administration may lead to volume overload. A urinary catheter to record urine output may be at risk of infection.

Endocrine: Medications and stress related to critical illness may worsen his glucose control.

Hematologic: Laboratory draws and volume administration may lead to anemia and potential need for transfusion.

Infectious disease (ID): Antibiotic administration may increase risk for antibiotic resistance and secondary infections after alteration of gut microbiome. He may be at risk of developing additional infections related to his central line and to the ventilator.

Musculoskeletal: He is at increased risk of progressive immobility and weakness. He may experience a loss in muscle mass and have progressive difficulty with recovery. This can be worsened in the setting of medications that can worsen myopathy (paralytics, steroids). Immobility may increase the risk of pressure ulcers and skin breakdown especially in the setting of suboptimal nutrition.

Social: Lack of access to familiar routines and loved ones may lead to depression. This may increase the risk of withdrawal and decreased desire to participate in care.

Will our patient develop all of these complications? Maybe not. In fact, many can be mitigated through attention to good, evidence-based critical care practices. Hopefully though, this list gives an appreciation of the risk that every patient experiences every day that they spend in our intensive care units. No wonder that we are so focused on getting people better and out of the ICU!

DOES ECMO FIX ALL THESE COMPLICATIONS?

Certainly not. In fact, patients on ECMO may be at higher risk of some of these complications – infections and bleeding immediately come to mind. However, two points should be underscored by this example.

First, the degree of benefit of ECMO is directly related to what toxicity we can mitigate. This is the degree that the slope can be flattened of the green line representing care on ECMO in our graph. If placing someone on ECMO will allow for a significant reduction in ventilator settings, sedation, pressor requirement, and facilitate ambulation, the benefit of ECMO will be much higher than if a less profound impact can be anticipated.

Second, and just as important, the principle of reducing toxicity should inform the day-to-day management of patients on ECMO. Whenever possible, ECMO should be used to facilitate the reduction of toxicity of care, for example, preferentially optimizing the ECMO circuit to ensure the maintenance of lung-protective settings. The more this can be done, the greater the derived benefit of ECMO support.

PUTTING IT TOGETHER

At its best, good ECMO management translates into excellent critical care. Good critical care management is not only a prerequisite for caring for a patient on ECMO, but can also be facilitated while on ECMO in a way that cannot be facilitated in conventional care.

Whenever possible, use the advantages of being on ECMO to facilitate recovery and to implement best practice care for your patient. You can optimize blood flow to the circuit to maximize oxygen delivery, in order for excess sedation, analgesia, and paralytics to be removed. You can increase the amount of support to allow for maximal performance with physical therapy. You can adjust sweep gas flow to allow for lung-protective mechanical ventilation settings.

As such, we will not be spending a lot of time reviewing best practices in this section. To your best ability, treat infections, optimize nutrition, facilitate rehabilitation, mitigate delirium, and engage family/surrogates to best treat the patient. Whenever possible, ECMO should be used to further implement rather than to impede these goals.

Rather, the remainder of this section will focus on the management aspects unique to the care of patients on ECMO – flow/sweep titration, anticoagulation, mechanical ventilation techniques, and pharmacokinetics. Let's now move ahead to further chapters to explore these unique attributes of management of patients on ECMO.

SUGGESTED READING

Lorusso, R., Shekar, K., MacLaren, G., Schmidt, M., Pellegrino, V., Meyns, B., et al. (2021). ELSO interim guidelines for venoarterial extracorporeal membrane oxygenation in adult cardiac patients. *ASAIO Journal, 67*(8), 827–844.

Tonna, J. E., Abrams, D., Brodie, D., Greenwood, J. C., Rubio Mateo-Sidron, J. A., Usman, A., et al. (2021). Management of adult patients supported with venovenous extracorporeal membrane oxygenation (VV ECMO): Guideline from the Extracorporeal Life Support Organization (ELSO). *ASAIO Journal, 67*(6), 601–610.

17

Blood Flow Titration

Imagine that you are initiating a patient on extracorporeal membrane oxygenation (ECMO). The cannulas are in excellent position and the circuit is connected and ready to go. You release the clamp and dark blood flows out smoothly.

"Time on ECMO, 7:38 a.m." you say.

Within a few seconds, bright red blood is infusing into the return cannula. You give a reassuring glance at the console – circuit pressures look good, flows are steady, everything is running well. Next, your eyes move to the monitor. The oxygen saturation begins to slowly improve, blood pressure is coming up, and the heart rate comes down.

As the cannulas are being secured and dressed, someone asks, "what settings should we start?"

Now comes the real challenge…

We will now get into the nuts and bolts of the daily management of ECMO. We have said again and again that ECMO really only involves the manipulation of a few variables, namely, sweep gas and blood flow. Now that you are armed with the physiologic principles at play, you can start to develop some management principles for how to titrate flow and sweep for your patients on ECMO.

THE INS AND OUTS OF FLOW TITRATION

Blood flow determines the amount of oxygen delivered by increasing the relative amount of oxygenated blood from the circuit relative to the overall output of the native heart and lungs. The higher the flow, the more oxygenated blood is being delivered to the body. Flow titration requires identification of the ideal amount of blood flow through the ECMO circuit required to meet the desired physiologic end points.

HOW MUCH FLOW IS ENOUGH? HOW MUCH IS TOO MUCH?

The ideal blood flow can be hard to define. While the individual physiologic needs and limits of the patient are the primary consideration, other considerations may come down to the style of the individual practitioners/programs. Needless to say, let's explore some principles that can be applied when trying to reach this flow.

As you increase flow, you will likely run into the following limits:

1. Minimum flow needed to maintain the pump
2. Achievement of a physiologic end point
3. You have reached a physiologic limit
4. You have reached a limit of the pump

Once you define these limits for each individual patient, you can better understand the ideal amount of flow to apply. Just because you *can* flow more doesn't mean you *should* flow more.

Limit #1: Minimum Flow Needed to Maintain the Pump

When you are first initiating ECMO, before the last clamp is released, there will be a minimum revolutions per minute (RPM) that is maintained, usually around 1500 RPM. Why is this? Why not just start at 0 and work your way up?

Remember when we were talking about the physiology of the pump, that forward flow is generated by the pressure differential from the pump. This pressure differential has to be enough to overcome the afterload of the pump, which comes in the form of the resistance of the circuit and either the mean arterial pressure (MAP) (in VA ECMO) or the central venous pressure (CVP) (in VV ECMO) (Fig. 17.1).

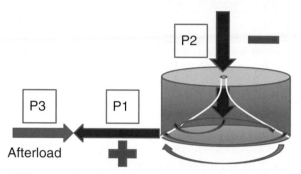

FIG. 17.1 The effect of afterload on pump function

At very low flows, the afterload may overtake the pressure generated by the pump at which you can have either no flow or retrograde flow. Additionally, the lower the flow, the greater the risk of stasis of blood and thrombosis in both the pump and in the oxygenator.

Put together, there is a minimum amount of blood flow that is maintained, usually no less than around 1.5 to 2 L in adults. Maintaining less flow may require a connection in the circuit separating the flow generated from the pump from the flow delivered to the patient (referred to as a bridge).

Limit #2: Achievement of a Physiologic Endpoint

Good critical care involves identifying a deficiency, applying an intervention, assessing the effect, and adjusting course. It is one thing to place a patient on fluids. It is much more effective to notice that a patient's labs, examination findings, and urine output are likely consistent with hypovolemia, give a bolus of fluid, and monitor the patient clinically to observe the clinical effect.

The same is true for flow, which is a form of support that can be dosed just like fluids, pressors, or mechanical ventilation. We spent a good deal of time in the ECMO Physiology section discussing and unpacking the physiologic rationale for ECMO, all of which are directly related to flow. Let's review:

Physiologic rational for ECMO
VV ECMO:
Clear CO_2
Mitigate shunt physiology
Optimize right heart function
VA ECMO:
Optimize perfusion
Support MAP
Perfuse visceral organs
Support right heart
Provide oxygenation

VV ECMO: Recall that VV ECMO improves oxygen by mitigating shunt physiology. In respiratory failure, as shunt increases, more blood passes from the right side of the heart to the left side without participating in gas exchange. As ECMO blood flow increases, it takes on a higher percentage of this total blood flow that is crossing the pulmonary circulation, and oxygenation improves. In a similar way, while sweep gas flow is the primary determinant of CO_2 clearance, recall from Chapter 11 that the higher the blood flow, the more CO_2 is cleared for every increase in sweep gas flow.

What does this mean for titration? The main take-home is that flow is related to DO_2. If there is evidence of inadequate DO_2 (low venous oxygen saturation, tachycardia, hypoxia), then this is where we have to evaluate for higher flow. The decision to consider at this point is increasing flow, tolerating lower DO_2, or giving blood.

VA ECMO: In Chapter 13, we talked about the vicious cycle of cardiogenic shock and how VA ECMO flow can help to mitigate these factors. Now is the time to titrate these effects. MAP is low? Lactate is not clearing fast enough? Urine output is borderline? CVP and PA pressures are increasing showing evidence that the right heart is straining? These are the clinical indicators that more blood flow may be needed.

Remember, flow is like a pressor or any other drug that must be titrated. Notice a deficiency, titrate the flow up or down, and then observe if this change achieved the target effect. Now we are getting somewhere!

Limit #3: You Have Reached a Physiologic/Anatomic Limit

At a certain point, flow starts to adversely impact the physiology of the patient. This can be subtle or very obvious and can overlap with the beneficial effects of increased flow as described earlier. As such, it may be difficult to compile a comprehensive list, but for the meantime, let's explore some adverse physiologic implications of too much flow.

Excessive negative venous pressure: Remember that to generate flow, the centrifugal pump generates a negative venous pressure, sucking blood out of the venous system through the pump. As flow increases this negative pressure grows, pulling the vena cava and the venous structures towards the cannula (Fig. 17.2).

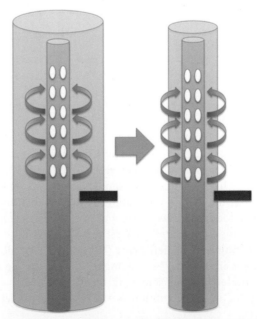

FIG. 17.2 Excessive negative pressure leading to collapse of the inferior vena cava

The effect of this can range anywhere from some mild kicking of the lines to dropping the flows for the circuit.

Biotrauma: Biotrauma refers to the inflammatory effect of support to tissues on a microscopic level. It is often described for mechanical ventilation, quantifying the damaging effects of mechanical ventilation that may be not accounted for by barotrauma and volutrauma effects alone. It is possible that higher blood flow through an artificial membrane oxygenator may lead to biotrauma as well, which can increase with increasing blood flow.

Recirculation (VV ECMO): This is a concept that we are now very familiar with but one that should be put in the context of flow titration. As flow increases on VV ECMO, there is more negative pressure generated by the drainage cannula, meaning there is a higher likelihood of pulling blood that is returning from the circuit back into the drainage cannula, as illustrated in Fig. 17.3. This has the dual effect of decreasing the effective ECMO blood flow and decreasing the efficiency of the membrane, by raising the saturation of blood entering the membrane.

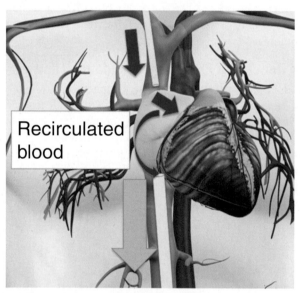

FIG. 17.3 Recirculation while on VV ECMO (Modified from SciePro/Shutterstock.com.)

What does this mean for flow titration? It means that as we increase blood flow, we need to look for evidence of recirculation, such as higher saturation of pre-oxygenator blood, a narrowing gap between pre-oxygenator O_2 saturation and patient O_2 saturation, and narrowing gap between pre-oxygenator CO_2 and post-oxygenator CO_2 levels.

Right ventricular and pulmonary vascular effects (VV ECMO): While on VV ECMO, the net flow of blood to the right atrium should be even – any blood that is returned to the heart is taken away from the venous circulation. However, there remains the possibility that the flow direction and velocity adversely affects the right ventricle and the pulmonary circulation. The overall adverse impact of this effect is yet to be defined.

Retrograde flow and the left heart (VA ECMO): We described the adverse effects of retrograde blood flow in Chapter 14. The higher the retrograde flow that is applied, the greater the afterload that the left heart must to work against. The heart's ability to accommodate this is largely influenced by the overall condition of the heart and the etiology causing the shock. This can manifest as decreased pulsatility, higher probability of ventricular/valvular thrombus, increasing workload and worsening ischemia, and pulmonary edema with worsening oxygenation.

Some of these effects can be readily observed and quantified at the bedside, while others may be less readily apparent or even theoretical. The effects and limits of increasing blood flow can exist as a spectrum as illustrated in Fig. 17.4.

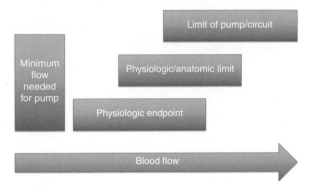

FIG. 17.4 Effects and limits of increasing blood flow

Does this mean that increasing blood flow is wrong at any given time? Not necessarily. What it does mean is that you should quantify the effect that you are aiming for and titrate flow to that effect. It is a subtle distinction, but one that will pay dividend if applied for your patients.

Limit #4: You Have Reached a Limit of the ECMO Pump/Circuit

Many of these limits have been explored in Chapter 10. To review:

Limit of the pump: The centrifugal pump generates forward flow by generating negative pressure on the drainage side and positive pressure on the return side. The greater the difference in these pressures, the greater the resulting flow will be. However, this is dependent on the speed of the pump – all pumps have a maximum amount of RPMs that they are able to generate. This is relevant to your patient because the higher the RPMs, the higher the probability that the pump speeds will be damaging to the blood that is crossing the pump.

There is no absolute number of RPMs that does or does not cause hemolysis, and this may change based on the configuration of the pump head/motor. Rather than aim for a specific number of RPMs, attempt to keep RPMs as low as possible to achieve the target flow (and more importantly target physiologic endpoint) and observe for evidence of hemolysis when RPMs are increased. If RPMs are being increased with a minimal increase in flow, this may be an indication that you are reaching the limits of the pump to increase flow.

Limit of the membrane: We introduced the concept of the rated flow of the membrane oxygenator – the flow at which no more oxygen transfer can occur. This is a standard value that is usually set by the manufacturer. Recall that as blood flow increases, the oxygen content transferred from the membrane increases, but at a decreasing rate. As flow increases, observe for evidence of diminishing returns by observing the oxygen levels of the post-oxygenator blood gas (Fig. 17.5).

Limit of the circuit/cannulas: The primary way the circuit/cannula limits flow is through resistance to flow, as described in our equation:

$$\text{Flow} = \frac{\pi \times \Delta P \times r^4}{8 \times \text{viscosity} \times \text{length}}$$

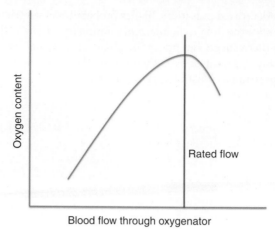

FIG. 17.5. Oxygenation capability of the oxygenator relative to blood flow

The narrower the cannulas and the longer the tubing, the more there will be resistance to flow. This will manifest as higher post-pump pressures and can eventually damage the circuit/oxygenator.

SEPARATING OUT PRELOAD FROM AFTERLOAD LIMITATIONS OF THE PUMP/CIRCUIT

We previously described the centrifugal pump as preload dependent and afterload sensitive. This means that preload is necessary for the pump to function and a lack of preload will rapidly drop the flow that the pump is able to generate. Afterload, on the other hand, will impact the overall flow of blood, dropping flow in proportion to the afterload that it must pump against.

Preload to the pump is determined by the intravascular volume of the venous system, size and compliance of the vena cava, pump speed, cannula size, and cannula position. The impact of cannula size and position is paramount, since it is often the variable that can be anticipated at selection. Larger diameter, multistage cannulas allow for more drainage of blood for any given speed of the pump and can allow for preload to the pump without excessive negative venous pressures. Cannula position can allow for adequate preload – a femoral drainage cannula placed in the intrahepatic inferior vena cava (IVC) can allow for drainage of blood with less vena caval collapse since the liver helps to stent the vena cava open.

Afterload to the pump, you will recall, is determined by resistance of the circuit/oxygenator/return cannula as well as the pressure of the system that blood is being returned to. For VV ECMO, this will be approximated by the CVP while for VA ECMO, this will be approximated by the MAP.

As a general principle, limitation to flow on VV ECMO will be on the negative side and is often due to the size of the drainage cannula while the limitation to flow on VA ECMO is more likely to be on the afterload side due to the return cannula.

This is not always the case. For example, there can be a lack of preload in VA ECMO, especially in the setting of hypovolemia/bleeding and VV ECMO can have excessive afterload, due to kinking of the lines, oxygenator clots, or coughing/clamping down. However, using this principle can allow for a system of what to evaluate first, when you encounter a drop in flow in a patient on VV versus VA ECMO.

Features to suggest a limitation of preload include excessive negative venous pressures, flow jumping up and down, and flow drops that improve with winding down the RPMs administering fluid. By contrast, flow that drops and stays down and flow that does not improve with decreasing RPMs/administering fluid may be more likely to be associated with afterload limitations to flow.

What This Means for the Patient on a Day-To-Day Basis

As you can see, there are many variables that go into what flow you are running on a day-to-day basis. This can get complex very quickly and can lead to uncertainty in the best way to support the patient.

We will apply our same critical care management principles to flow – identify a deficiency, apply an intervention, assess the effect, and adjust course. When it comes to ECMO blood flow, try to identify what goals you are trying to accomplish with any flow, assess if those goals are being met, and what limits are holding you back.

> For the most part, if the same physiologic endpoint can be achieved with a lower flow, go with the lower flow. Just because you can flow higher doesn't necessarily mean that you should flow higher.

This principle will serve well to limit any damaging effects of high blood flow and can potentially limit biotrauma. Additionally, it will allow for the natural progression to weaning, as detailed later.

WEANING ECMO BLOOD FLOW

As heart and lung recovery progresses, the ability of the body to adequately deliver oxygen improves to the point that ECMO may no longer be necessary, allowing for ECMO to be weaned off. This can be one of the most fulfilling parts of the care of any patient on ECMO. As the physiology of VV and VA ECMO is very different, we will discuss the strategies and rationale for weaning each separately.

Blood Flow Weaning and VV ECMO

As the lungs begin to improve, there is more participation of the alveolar unit in gas exchange. This leads to more V:Q matching and a lower shunt fraction. Now all of a sudden, blood that is pumped out of the right heart across the pulmonary circulation is not completely shunted across.

The result is the reverse of the process that we uncovered when we discussed respiratory failure – less intrapulmonary shunt means less blood flow from the ECMO circuit that is needed to capture the cardiac output. This will mean that you will be able to achieve physiologic endpoints of improved oxygen delivery (limit #2 above) without running into a limit from the ECMO pump or an anatomic/physiologic limit (limit #3 and #4 above).

However, at a certain point, you begin to reach the limit of what the pump needs to run. For some pumps this will be 3 L, for some 2.5 L or even lower. Regardless, there will be a point when lowering blood flow will not be sufficient to determine whether the patient is able to wean from VV ECMO. At this point, you must rely on sweep weaning (see Chapter 18).

Blood Flow Weaning and VA ECMO

Weaning ECMO blood flow is the primary mechanism of weaning for VA ECMO. As opposed to VV ECMO, which still relies on the ability of the right/left heart to provide cardiac output for oxygen delivery, overall perfusion is the sum of the native cardiac output and the flow from the machine, as follows:

$$CO_{ECMO} = Native\ CO + ECMO\ blood\ flow$$

Therefore, to truly understand the ability of the native heart and lungs, flow must be weaned down or even off briefly. The actual blood flow that can be tolerated for weaning will vary depending on the risk of clotting, the overall status of the patient, and the individual protocols of the institution. A patient with complete cardiac recovery and a robust MAP will likely need a much shorter weaning trial than a patient with borderline cardiac function.

Variables that can be accounted for while assessing the ability to wean include the following:
- **Vital signs:** MAP, heart rate
- **PA catheter pressures:** PA systolic, PA diastolic, CVP pulmonary capillary wedge pressure
- **Echocardiogram findings:** left ventricular function, right ventricular function, aortic valve opening, etc.
- **Clinical evidence of perfusion:** urine output, mental status, capillary refill
- **Laboratory findings:** venous oxygen saturation, lactic acid

The lower the flows (less than 2 L/min, for example) and the longer the amount of time needed for the weaning trial (hours v. minutes), the greater the risk of thrombus in the cannula, oxygenator, or circuit. Higher anticoagulation targets may be needed.

Why Can You Wean Flow to Assess for Weaning VA ECMO But Not for VV ECMO?

Let's summarize the difference in weaning blood flows in VV versus VA ECMO:

> **Weaning and VV/VV ECMO**
> **VV ECMO:** Flows may be weaned to a point where physiologic endpoints are met but not to assess for separation from support. To assess for removal, wean **sweep**
> **VA ECMO:** Flow must be weaned to assess for ability to remove ECMO

The reason VV ECMO flows cannot be weaned to assess for decannulation is because the time period for weaning is often on the order of hours, which could be poorly tolerated with increased risk of thrombus and pump stoppage. Additionally, native CO_2 clearance is often slow to normalize in respiratory failure as compared to cardiac failure, meaning that sweep weaning will be a truer test of ability to wean rather than blood flow wean. We will go into sweep gas titration/weaning in more detail in the next chapter.

In VA ECMO, the contribution of ECMO blood flow to the overall perfusion is the main indication for support. If clinical endpoints can be met with low to no flow, then there is a high likelihood of successfully being able to separate from support and decannulate.

Now that we have a much better sense of how to titrate blood flow, we will now move into principles for titration of sweep gas flow.

SUGGESTED READING

Shekar, K., Buscher, H., & Brodie, D. (2020). Protocol-driven daily optimisation of venovenous extracorporeal membrane oxygenation blood flows: an alternate paradigm? *Journal of Thoracic Disease*, *12*(11), 6854.

Keller, S. P. (2019). Management of peripheral venoarterial extracorporeal membrane oxygenation in cardiogenic shock. *Critical Care Medicine*, *47*(9), 1235.

Burkhoff, D., Sayer, G., Doshi, D., & Uriel, N. (2015). Hemodynamics of mechanical circulatory support. *Journal of the American College of Cardiology*, *66*(23), 2663–2674.

18

Sweep Gas Flow Titration

Adjustments to sweep gas flow are probably the most common adjustments that you will make in the course of an extracorporeal membrane oxygenation (ECMO) run. While it is entirely feasible that you can go for days on the same blood flow, sweep may need to be adjusted on a daily basis or even multiple times per day.

There is little evidence on optimal strategies for sweep titration and there is significant variation in practice patterns. That said, having a structured approach to adjusting sweep can shape the course of the ECMO run and can optimize management of patients on ECMO. As such, the strategies presented should not be taken as definitive but rather as a proposed approach to the physiologic principles at play.

In general, sweep gas titration is a skill set that gets better with practice. Every adjustment that is made to sweep parameters is an opportunity to assess the clinical impact. As with all critical care interventions, you should have a rationale for changes, estimate the expected result, and then reassess the clinical response. This approach will hone your intuition and serve to refine your clinical thought processes. Remember, practice doesn't make perfect, perfect practice makes perfect.

BASICS OF SWEEP GAS FLOW TITRATION

Recall that the oxygenator membrane is semi-permeable, allowing for O_2 and CO_2 to diffuse down their respective concentration gradients and that while both molecules are able to move across the membrane, the diffusibility of CO_2 is six times greater than the diffusibility of O_2 (Fig. 18.1).

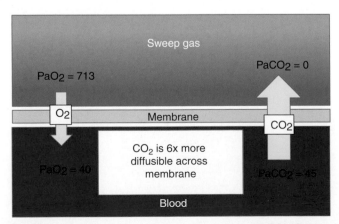

FIG. 18.1 Relative diffusibility of CO_2 v. O_2 across the ECMO membrane

This higher diffusibility of CO_2 means that the rate of gas flow directly correlates with how fast CO_2 is cleared. The higher the rate of gas flow, the faster CO_2 is removed from the blood.

This concept underlies the convention provided that **$PaCO_2$** is primarily affected by adjustments to **flow rate of sweep gas**, while **PaO_2** of the blood leaving the oxygenator is primarily affected by adjustments to the **FiO_2** of the sweep gas flow (Fig. 18.2).

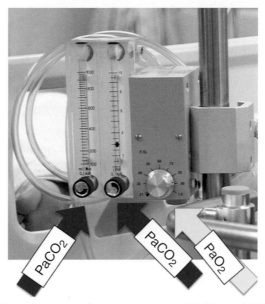

FIG. 18.2 Manipulate sweep gas flow rate to control $PaCO_2$ and FiO_2 to control PaO_2. (From PIJITRA PHOMKHAM/Shutterstock.com.)

For the most part, adjustments of 1 L or greater should be made with the middle knob (increments of 0.5 L) while adjustments to sweep of <1 L should be made with the knob on the left (increments of 100mL), to allow for more precise titration. These two knobs will be additive, so that if the middle knob is set to 4 L/min and the left knob is set to 500 mL/min, the patient will be receiving 4.5 L/min of sweep gas flow.

How much does an adjustment in sweep gas flow affect $PaCO_2$ of arterial blood? The answer lies in the efficiency of the membrane oxygenator, the presence of recirculation, minute ventilation

> As a general rule of thumb, an increase in sweep gas flow by 1 L/min can be expected to decrease $PaCO_2$ by 5–10 mmHg.

and dead space of the native lungs, and the CO_2 gradient, which is a function of $PaCO_2$ entering into the membrane oxygenator via the venous blood.

The presence of the aforementioned mitigating factors requires that adjustments to sweep gas flow are put into the correct clinical context. Whenever possible, confirm the result of changes in sweep by monitoring the clinical response of the patient (dyspnea, tachypnea, apnea, encephalopathy, etc.) as well as the patient arterial blood gas when clinically appropriate.

PLACING SWEEP GAS FLOW INTO THE CLINICAL PHASE OF ECMO SUPPORT

"Easy enough, when CO_2 is high, go up on sweep and when CO_2 is low go down on sweep, right?" While this is sometimes the case, there is often more subtlety to the titration of sweep gas flow.

The first consideration is what phase of ECMO support the patient is in. While the clinical characteristics of an ECMO run can vary, with setbacks and improvements throughout, we can expect an overall pattern involving three distinct phases: stabilization, maintenance, and weaning. The way we adjust and titrate sweep gas flow will differ significantly depending on what phase we are in. Let's use the graph in Fig. 18.3 to illustrate.

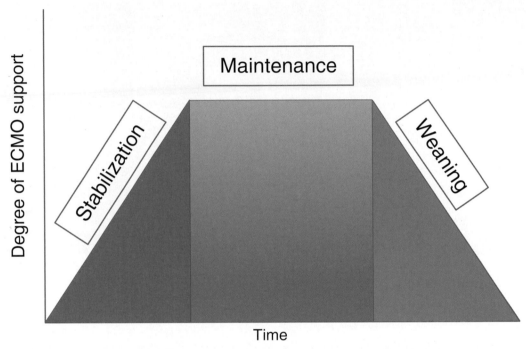

FIG. 18.3 Placing sweep gas flow adjustments into the context of the phase of ECMO support

Stabilization: Stabilization is the period where we are trying to manage and mitigate end organ damage. We are trying to prevent the vicious cycle of cardiac and respiratory failure that could lead to multiorgan failure, with progressive and sequential shutdown of peripheral tissue beds.

During this period, sweep gas flow titration tends to be much more aggressive, with an emphasis on correcting acidosis as well as CO_2 in order to optimize right ventricular afterload, cerebral perfusion, as well as perfusion to end organ tissue beds.

When initiating ECMO, the common convention is to initiate sweep at a 1:1 rate with blood flow and adjust thereafter based on clinical/laboratory parameters. As an example, if you initiate ECMO and the blood flow is set to 3 L/min, sweep gas can be set to 3 L/min with the plan to check arterial blood gases 20–30 minutes after initiating ECMO.

Maintenance: This is the period where stabilization has occurred but the patient still needs ECMO support. The focus of the overall management shifts from mitigating further decompensation to advancing rehabilitation, optimizing nutrition, weaning sedation, and preventing and managing complications.

The length of this period may range from days to weeks depending on the level of support and the overall course of disease.

Sweep gas flow targets in this phase are aimed towards maintaining lung-protective/ultra–lung-protective ventilation, preventing encephalopathy, and patient comfort by titrating to prevent dyspnea/apnea.

When it comes to sweep gas in this phase, there is a rationale/advantage for parsimony. If the patient is not clinically impacted, uncomfortable, or encephalopathic, and if lung-protective ventilation is maintained, maintaining less sweep allows for the ability to increase when needed and allows for engagement of the lungs in CO_2 clearance. Similar to our discussion with blood flow titration, just because you *can* flow at a higher sweep does not mean you *should* flow higher.

Weaning: This is often the most gratifying phase. As the heart/lungs improve, dead space decreases, and V/Q mismatch improves. Additionally, fluid is mobilized from the pulmonary interstitium into the intravascular space, with improved pulmonary compliance, better minute ventilation, and more CO_2 clearance from the native lungs.

This is the phase where sweep can be weaned more aggressively, allowing the lungs to take on more of the load of CO_2 clearance. Sweep can be downtitrated if patient is in the weaning phase, even if the $PaCO_2$ is normal or even modestly elevated.

Confirm that you are truly in the weaning phase by assessing as many clinical variables as you can. Some questions to ask include:

- Is the compliance on the ventilator improving?
- Is the chest X-ray clear/improved?
- Is there evidence of heart/lung recovery in terms of oxygenation (improved PaO_2)?
- Is there evidence of mobilization of fluid with increased urine output and net negative fluid balance despite minimal or stable diuretics?
- Has blood flow been decreased with minimal impact on clinical status?

As more and more of these scenarios become true, the assumption that the heart/lungs are recovering becomes an increasingly reasonable proposition.

However, note that this can only be done if the patient is truly improved and the lungs are ready to take on the burden of increased CO_2 clearance. If not, this can lead to injury to the lungs, especially if weaning requires a significant escalation in ventilator settings. Patience is paramount – the heart/lungs will take over when they are ready.

IMPACT OF SWEEP GAS FLOW ON CO_2 BUFFERING

CO_2 dissolves in water to form carbonic acid, which dissociates to bicarbonate/hydrogen ion based on the following equilibrium:

$$H_2O + CO_2 \rightleftharpoons H^+CO^+ \rightleftharpoons HCO_3^- + H^+$$

This equilibrium means that excess CO_2 will lead to acidosis in the acute phase, but this acid can be buffered out over time as kidneys resorb HCO_3^-. This process allows for two phenomena, which are beneficial to the patient with difficulty with CO_2 clearance:

1. Mitigates acidosis from excessive CO_2 through resorption of bicarbonate
2. Allows for two mechanisms to remove CO_2 from the body: lungs (CO_2) and kidneys (HCO_3^-)

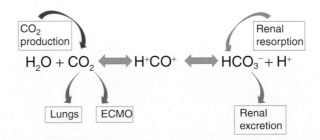

While resorption of excess bicarbonate can take years to accumulate in the case of chronic respiratory acidosis due to chronic obstructive pulmonary disease (COPD) or obstructive sleep apnea, bicarbonate resorption can occur over the course of days in the ICU, particularly in the case of respiratory acidosis due to severe heart/lung failure requiring ECMO.

Therefore, the effect of bicarbonate buffering should be taken into account while adjusting sweep gas flow CO_2. Let's examine how this manifests clinically.

Adjusting Sweep for pH Versus $PaCO_2$

If bicarbonate is high due to elevated CO_2 levels, normalizing the $PaCO_2$ can have the adverse effect of inducing a metabolic alkalosis. This may equilibrate eventually, but there can be adverse effects of changing the CO_2 levels before the patient can adjust. By adjusting sweep gas flow based on the pH rather than the $PaCO_2$, you will allow for adjustments in $PaCO_2$ that are within the set point for the patient.

This convention is typically employed for the maintenance phase. In the resuscitation phase, when there is the possibility of end organ decompensation, normal CO_2 may be targeted in order to prevent cerebral vasodilation/vasoconstriction or to minimize pulmonary vascular resistance/right ventricular afterload.

Adjusting Sweep When pH Is Normal and $PaCO_2$/Bicarbonate Is High

Let's consider the case of a patient with worsening CO_2 clearance from the lungs who may also have increasing CO_2 production due to infection, sepsis, or general critical illness. This patient will have elevated total body CO_2 content, with elevated CO_2 as well as HCO_3^- levels, and a consequent normal pH. Increasing sweep alone may lead to metabolic alkalosis. One strategy involves lowering HCO_3^- levels by allowing for dumping of HCO_3^- with a drug like acetazolamide and increasing sweep gas flow if the patient becomes acidotic. The utility of this strategy will depend on the renal function of the patient and an assessment on whether a potential rise in CO_2 will be well tolerated clinically.

Either way, total body CO_2 as a function of $PaCO_2$ and HCO_3^- needs to be accounted for when making adjustments to sweep gas flow.

SWEEP GAS TITRATION AT THE BEDSIDE

You may be getting a sense of the complexity related to adjustments in sweep gas flow. You may adjust sweep gas very differently for a patient placed on VA ECMO due to cardiac arrest 24 hours ago who is at risk for cerebral edema than a patient on VV ECMO for viral pneumonia who is 40 days into his ECMO run and with a clearing CXR. Whenever possible, place decisions on sweep titration into the context of the total CO_2 burden, to include $PaCO_2$ and HCO_3^- in addition to the clinical phase of illness. Below is a summary of factors to consider based on the phase of support.

Phase of ECMO support	Reason for sweep increase	Reason for sweep decrease
Stabilization	• Normalize pH and $PaCO_2$ (optimizing right ventricle and cerebral circulation) • Avoid tachypnea/ dyspnea to whatever extent possible	• Avoid hypocarbia • Alkalotic with normal/ low $PaCO_2$
Maintenance	• Rest lungs/minimize ventilator settings • Respiratory acidosis • Adverse effects of CO_2: encephalopathy, tachypnea • Worsening oxygenator performance • Normalize bicarbonate	• Respiratory alkalosis • Prevent apnea • Engage lungs in ventilation
Weaning	• Fails weaning trial • Weaned sweep too fast	• Alkalosis or normal pH • Challenge lungs

SWEEP GAS TITRATION IN VA ECMO

The principles outlined earlier apply to VV and VA ECMO, as they dictate the amount of CO_2 clearance that is facilitated by the oxygenator and how this will be translated into the $PaCO_2$ of blood returning to the body.

Clearly, the way this blood interacts with the body differs between VV ECMO and VA ECMO and should be considered when making adjustments.

VA ECMO allows for the blood to flow directly into the arterial circulation. The effect of this convention is that sweep gas flow is generally weaned much more quickly on VA ECMO support. It is not uncommon to rapidly wean down sweep gas flow to 1 L/min or 0.5 L/min for a patient on VA ECMO.

In fact, patients on minimal sweep (say 0.5 L/min) may continue to have a respiratory alkalosis with a low $PaCO_2$ and elevated pH. The temptation may be to wean sweep gas flow to off. However, **do not wean sweep gas flow off on VA ECMO!** Doing so will take deoxygenated blood from the venous circulation and dump it into the arterial circulation resulting in a rapid decompensation.

Weaning is generally done differently in VV versus VA ECMO. Let's examine the primary strategies for each.

WEANING IN VA ECMO

Recall that VA ECMO provides direct support for cardiac output in an additive fashion, where overall perfusion provided is the sum of native cardiac output and ECMO blood flow.

Assessment of readiness to wean from VA ECMO involves the ability to wean blood flow. Blood flow can be weaned at bedside in a patient with complete recovery or over the course of days in patients with a more uncertain recovery. The risks of slower wean (longer period at low flows, higher risk of thrombosis) should be weighed against the benefits (more gradual weaning, higher certainty of ability to successfully wean) (Fig. 18.4).

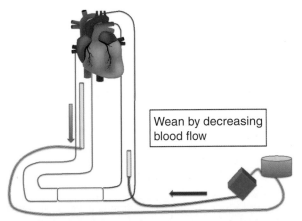

Wean by decreasing blood flow

FIG. 18.4 Weaning on VA ECMO: decrease blood flow while maintaining some sweep gas flow. (Modified from Ody_Stocker/Shutterstock.com.)

After weaning down blood flow to a minimal level (say 1.5 L/min to 2.5 L/min), the ECMO circuit is sometimes clamped to examine the effect of cessation of blood flow. This can only be done for a brief period as static blood can increase the risk of thrombosis and embolization.

Sweep gas flow should be weaned down to a minimal level prior to weaning off ECMO. The maintenance of some sweep gas flow is absolutely necessary, and titrating off sweep gas flow completely will deoxygenate any blood flow that is going through the ECMO circuit. Even though it was already mentioned, it is an essential point, so indulge me.

> Never wean off sweep gas flow completely on VA ECMO. Doing so will lead to rapid decompensation.

Ok, now I'm satisfied.

WEANING IN VV ECMO

As opposed to VA ECMO, perfusion to end organs on VV ECMO is maintained completely by the native cardiac output. Therefore, the effect of weaning ECMO blood flow is less impactful in informing whether the patient is ready to be weaned. Blood flow may be able to be titrated up or down throughout the course as mentioned in the previous chapter, but the true test of whether the patient is ready to come off VV ECMO is ultimately the ability to wean off sweep gas flow (Fig. 18.5).

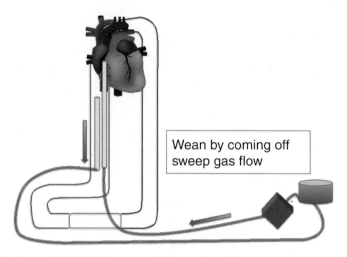

Wean by coming off sweep gas flow

FIG. 18.5 Weaning on VV ECMO: come off sweep gas flow completely while maintaining ECMO blood flow. (Modified from Ody_Stocker/Shutterstock.com.)

The advantage of maintaining ECMO blood flow while trialing off sweep gas involves getting a sense of what the patient is likely to look like off ECMO since any oxygenation/CO_2 clearance will be completely due to the performance of the native lungs. Additionally, since the blood flow through the ECMO circuit is maintained, longer trial periods can be maintained to examine the effect of weaning over the course of hours if needed.

The first thing to look for while weaning is oxygen saturation. While the patient may tolerate minimal sweep and appears ready to be weaned off ECMO, it is important to realize that the oxygenation of blood is maintained as long as any sweep gas is present. Turning off the sweep gas may lead to a drastic change if the patient is not ready to come off ECMO. This usually manifests as an acute drop in oxygen saturation within the first couple of minutes after sweep gas flow is turned off.

If oxygen saturation is maintained, the next variable to assess is work of breathing. A patient may be able to maintain oxygenation but may be tachypneic/dyspneic/fatigued in order to do so. This clinical constellation often means that the patient is improving but not yet ready to wean.

If a patient is able to maintain adequate oxygen saturation with a normal work of breathing, the final variable to monitor is CO_2 level. The ability to clear CO_2 sometimes lags behind the ability to oxygenate; therefore elevated $PaCO_2$ levels on ABG that cannot be optimized with lung-protective strategies may indicate a failure to wean.

The decision to wean must be weighed against the risks and benefits of staying on ECMO. Patients with complications related to ECMO (bleeding, infection, cannula issues) may warrant more aggressive weaning from ECMO.

That said, one final note about weaning on VV ECMO. Due to longer ECMO run times, the temptation may exist to push weaning in order to get a patient off ECMO. If not limited by complications, weaning often happens when the patient is ready to come off. Patience is key.

WEANING FiO$_2$ TO SWEEP GAS FLOW

We mentioned that FiO_2 is the final variable that can be manipulated with regards to sweep gas flow. Often this is set at 100% and left at 100% until the patient is able to be weaned off entirely.

FiO_2 can be weaned when PaO_2 of the arterial blood gas is high ($PaO_2 > 120$ mmHg), as hyperoxia can potentially be toxic. However, for the most part, while on ECMO support, PaO_2 is either low or normal. Weaning FiO_2 to sweep gas flow should be avoided if this means increasing the amount of oxygen administered to the native lungs, which often comes at a greater cost of toxicity.

The presence of high PaO_2 on the arterial blood gas is more likely to occur on VA ECMO, particularly when central cannulated. Adjustments in FiO_2 to sweep gas flow are more common in this mode of support.

Rarely, FiO_2 can be weaned as a last phase of weaning on VV ECMO, particularly in patients who are on minimal sweep gas flow, but who do not tolerate the final step off of trial completely off sweep. FiO_2 weaning in these patients may allow for a more gradual weaning in this select group of patients.

PUTTING IT TOGETHER

Some aspects of ECMO care are relatively consistent across different teams and programs, while other aspects involve practices that vary widely. The interpretation of CO_2 clearance, adjustment of sweep gas flow, and practices for weaning ECMO definitely fall into the latter category. Different teams and providers may employ different techniques for adjustment and titration of sweep gas flow – some making large changes with frequent adjustments while others employ a very conservative approach.

Ultimately, the right technique is that which leads to a good clinical response and ultimately a good outcome to the patient. Whenever possible, assess the clinical effect of changes in sweep gas flow. This will not only allow you to hone your skills of sweep gas flow titration but also contextualize your changes to a meaningful outcome for the patient under your care.

SUGGESTED READING

Aissaoui, N., Luyt, C. E., Leprince, P., Trouillet, J. L., Léger, P., & Pavie, A., et al. (2011). Predictors of successful extracorporeal membrane oxygenation (ECMO) weaning after assistance for refractory cardiogenic shock. *Intensive Care Medicine*, 37(11), 1738–1745.

Kenrick, B., de Vries, A. P. J., & Gans, R. O. B. (2014). Physiological approach to assessment of acid–base disturbances. *New England Journal of Medicine*, 371(15), 1434–1445.

Grant, A. A., Hart, V. J., Lineen, E. B., Badiye, A., Byers, P. M., & Patel, A., et al. (2018). A weaning protocol for venovenous extracorporeal membrane oxygenation with a review of the literature. *Artificial Organs*, *42*(6), 605–610.

Schmidt, M., Tachon, G., Devilliers, C., Muller, G., Hekimian, G., & Bréchot, N., et al. (2013). Blood oxygenation and decarboxylation determinants during venovenous ECMO for respiratory failure in adults. *Intensive Care Medicine*, *39*(5), 838–846.

19

Ventilator Management on ECMO

By this point you have probably developed a healthy skepticism for the ventilator. While remaining an undeniable cornerstone in the support of critically ill patients, we have gone into the myriad of limitations the ventilator has in severe respiratory failure, when compliance worsens and it becomes progressively difficult to oxygenate/ventilate.

Now we will progress to some principles for management of the ventilator while on extracorporeal membrane oxygenation (ECMO). It should be noted that this is one of the areas where there is probably the most variation in practice patterns, with some practitioners being very conservative with ventilator weaning, and others being very aggressive. Rather than advocating one approach over the other, we will try to focus this chapter on principles that can be applied in order to minimize the damaging effects of the ventilator for patients on ECMO. This will not be a comprehensive overview of all strategies of mechanical ventilation, but rather a very focused review of principles that are commonly applied to patients on ECMO.

We will focus this discussion on patients with primary respiratory failure, however the principles discussed will apply to all types of support.

COMMON VENTILATOR SETTINGS IN ECMO SUPPORT

Imagine you are caring for a patient who was just initiated on ECMO. As support was initiated, they had a phenomenal response – their saturations increased from 77% to 100%, their heartrate decreased from 120 to 98, and their blood pressure improved from 89/55 to 105/70.

Your eyes now turn to the ventilator. It reads as follows:

> Mode AC/VC. Tidal Volume 500. 100% FiO_2. PEEP 14. Rate 34. Peak pressures measured at 42.

Just as you are pondering the ventilator and the settings that you can transition this patient to, the respiratory therapist asks, "Do you want me to change the patient to our typical vent settings?" She then makes the following changes to the ventilator.

> Mode AC/PC. Inspiratory pressure 12. 50% FiO_2. PEEP 10. Rate 26. Tidal volume measured at 145 mL.

What is the difference between these two settings? What is the rationale behind these changes?

MODE OF VENTILATION: SPONTANEOUS VERSUS CONTROLLED VENTILATION

The mechanism of the ventilator is relatively straightforward – it pushes a set amount of air into the lungs. As such, you can imagine that there really are three primary variables that effect how this air is delivered: what initiates the breath (referred to as **trigger**), what is delivered with each breath (referred to as **limit**), and what ends the breath (referred to as **cycle**).

If the ventilator is delivering a set number of breaths regardless of whether the patient is initiating the breath or not, this is controlled ventilation. Contrast this to spontaneous ventilation, where every breath that is taken has to be initiated by the patient (Figs. 19.1 and 19.2).

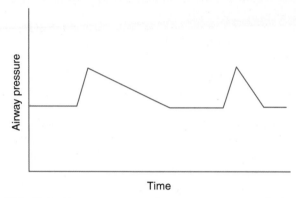

FIG. 19.1 Airway pressures in spontaneous ventilation

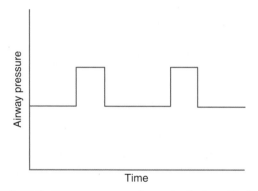

FIG. 19.2 Airway pressure in controlled ventilation

The other difference between these two modes is how the breath ends. In spontaneous mode, as you can see earlier, the breath can be long or short and is only stopped when a specific flow has been obtained. Compare this to controlled ventilation, in which the breath is stopped after a set amount of time. This may result in more variation in the size of the breath for spontaneous ventilation, which is similar to how we breathe without the ventilator, but may or may not be well tolerated in the setting of severe lung dysfunction.

In spontaneous ventilation, a certain amount of positive end-expiratory pressure (PEEP) is set followed by a set amount of pressure that is delivered above PEEP with every breath. The volume of breath that is generated is dependent on the flow that the patient is able to generate, based on the strength of the diaphragm.

This reliance on the diaphragm forms the main advantages and disadvantages of spontaneous ventilation. On one hand, this mode can condition the diaphragm, employing it in every breath similar to breathing without the ventilator. However, if there is severe decompensation, this may lead to overexertion and weakness.

How do you make the distinction between selecting spontaneous versus controlled ventilation? This is a challenging question to answer due to the wide range of approaches taken by various practitioners, as well as the varied response that individual patients can have. As a general rule, controlled ventilation may be needed early in the course, with the aim of allowing for spontaneous ventilation as the patient continues to wake up and recover. This can be over the course of several days or several hours, depending on how the patient is responding to weaning. Wean as much as is tolerated clinically.

What happens when spontaneous breathing is not feasible clinically? Let's go over a couple of considerations for controlled ventilation.

Controlled Ventilation: Volume Versus Pressure Control

The two main modes for controlled ventilation are pressure control and volume control. The difference between the two is as follows:

Volume control: delivers a set amount of **volume** with each controlled breath (flow limited/volume cycled)

Pressure control: delivers a set amount of **pressure** with each controlled breath (pressure limited/time cycled)

Minimizing both pressure and volume delivered is ideal, since as you remember, both can cause damage to the lungs in the form of barotrauma (pressure) and volutrauma (volume). The challenge comes when compliance decreases, as occurs when lungs get progressively stiff due to edema, acute respiratory distress syndrome (ARDS), pneumonia, hemorrhage, or any of the host of conditions that are associated with severe cardiac/respiratory failure. In this case, you are left with either tolerating higher pressures or lower tidal volumes, as denoted below:

$$\downarrow \text{Compliance} = \frac{V_T}{PIP - PEEP} \left< \begin{array}{l} \downarrow V_T \\ \uparrow P_{IP} \end{array} \right.$$

This is the tradeoff that often has to occur with worsening respiratory failure that leads to a failure to ventilate: either you have to tolerate higher CO_2 levels due to lower tidal volumes or you have to tolerate higher airway pressures in order to achieve a target tidal volume.

ECMO obviates the need for this choice. Since the circuit is able to remove CO_2 with great efficiency, you can significantly lower both the pressure and volume delivered with each breath and afford better lung protection from the damaging effects of barotrauma and volutrauma.

Either mode is acceptable as long as you are providing lung-protective ventilation.

Lung Protective Variable #1: Tidal Volume

Tidal volume is one of the mechanical ventilation parameters with the most well-established association to improved outcomes. We know that high tidal volumes are damaging to the lung parenchyma and that this damage has been linked to a higher mortality.

The generally accepted target is 6 mL per kg of ideal body weight. When compared to higher tidal volumes, tidal volumes of less that 6 mL/kg have been associated with improved mortality. What about 5 mL/kg? 4 mL/kg? 2 mL/kg?

6 mL/kg is usually the target because lower tidal volumes often leads to difficulty in removing CO_2, due to lower minute ventilation (tidal volume × breaths per minute). However, CO_2 removal is less of an issue in ECMO, allowing for lower tidal volumes if desired.

Thus, many practitioners aim for tidal volumes on ECMO less than **4 mL/kg**. This is sometimes referred to as "ultra–lung-protective ventilation." There is some evidence to support this strategy, as 4 mL/kg was the lower limit of normal in many trials.

Lung Protective Variable #2: Driving Pressure

Let's introduce this concept of driving pressure. Driving pressure is defined as follows:

Driving pressure = Plateau Pressure − PEEP

Driving pressure is not discussed as much as tidal volume, but actually has a higher association with improved outcomes.

Before we discuss driving pressure, let's examine what is meant by plateau pressure.

Recall in our discussion of flow dynamics, we used the example of two balloons connected by a plastic tube. We noted that the flow of air between the balloons is determined by the pressure difference between these balloons as well as the resistance of the tube. We used this example to illustrate the limits to blood flow through the ECMO circuit. Now let's apply this dynamic to the flow of air from the ventilator to the lungs (Fig. 19.3).

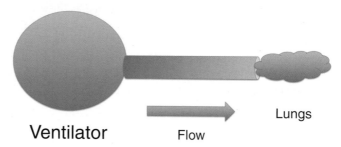

FIG. 19.3 Airway pressure and ventilation

In this case, there is a specific amount of pressure that has to be delivered to inflate the lungs based on the compliance of the lungs, but also a specific amount of pressure that has to be delivered to overcome the resistance of everything that connects the ventilator and the alveoli (such as the ventilator circuit, the endotracheal tube, the trachea, and the bronchi).

These two pressures can be differentiated by doing an inspiratory breath hold, which will measure the pressure required to distend the alveoli only as the resistance of the circuit is already overcome, known as the plateau pressure. Let's compare differences in plateau pressures for two patients with an elevated peak pressure. If there is minimal resistance in the connection, then the plateau pressure will be close to the peak pressure (blue line). On the other hand, if there is high resistance in the connection (due to kinking of the endotracheal tube, mucous plugging in the trachea, or spasm in the bronchi as examples), then the plateau pressure will be much lower than the peak pressure, as noted by the red line (Fig. 19.4).

The difference between the PEEP and the plateau pressure, as measured by an inspiratory breath hold, is the driving pressure. As a general rule, the lower the driving pressure the better. This can be accomplished by lowering the plateau pressure (through lower inspiratory pressures

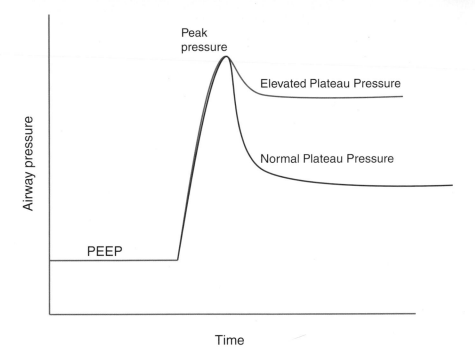

FIG. 19.4 Comparison of elevated plateau pressure (blue line) v. normal plateau pressure (red line). PEEP, Positive end-expiratory pressure

on pressure control or lower tidal volumes on volume control) or by increasing the PEEP. A driving pressure of **less than 10–15 cm H₂O** is a good target.

If increasing PEEP does not lead to a higher plateau pressure, this indicates lung recruitment and has been associated with a better outcome. Let's now discuss PEEP.

POSITIVE END-EXPIRATORY PRESSURE TARGETS DURING ECMO

PEEP is the minimum amount of positive pressure maintained by the ventilator, defined as the pressure at the end of expiration, as illustrated in Fig. 19.5. At a basic level, there are several benefits to maintaining some PEEP:
1. Prevents total alveolar collapse allowing for a specified number of alveoli to remain open
2. Facilitates improved oxygenation by raising mean airway pressure due to higher time spent in the expiratory phase
3. Allows for convective ventilation by keeping more alveoli open and participating in gas exchange
4. Improves hemodynamics by decreasing cardiac afterload

Too little PEEP can be detrimental; however, excessive PEEP can have an adverse effect by a host of mechanisms including:
1. Overdistension of alveoli, increasing the proportion of alveoli with dead space ventilation
2. Eventually raising plateau pressure, leading to barotrauma
3. Decreasing preload to right heart
4. Increasing right ventricular afterload

Finding the right amount of PEEP is key. One way to assess for ideal PEEP is to observe the effect of adjustments in PEEP to the patient. If increasing PEEP leads to improved hemodynamics,

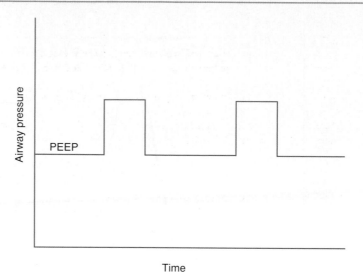

FIG. 19.5 PEEP and overall airway pressure. *PEEP,* Positive end-expiratory pressure

no change in plateau pressure, and better oxygenation, then this is an indicator that this change is well tolerated.

By convention, PEEP of **8–15 cm H$_2$O** is a reasonable starting target for patients on ECMO. Adjustments should be made thereafter based on the response of the patient.

LIMITING FiO$_2$ FROM THE VENTILATOR

Limiting FiO$_2$ from the ventilator is essential to prevent damage to the patient, but doing so takes a great deal of discipline. This is because patients on ECMO are often hypoxic, and it is difficult to see the harmful effects of high oxygen levels. In reality, high levels of FiO$_2$ can make it very difficult for lungs to improve. Let's explore the harm that can come from prolonged exposure to 100% FiO$_2$.

As we discussed in Chapter 5, when we normally breathe room air, only around 21% of the air we are breathing is oxygen. The rest is predominantly nitrogen (N$_2$), for which there does not exist the same diffusion gradient between the air in the alveoli and the blood as exists for O$_2$. As a result, the nitrogen that enters the alveoli remains in the alveoli for the most part. This nitrogen plays a key role in keeping the alveoli open.

Oxygen, on the other hand, is a key component of metabolism; therefore the blood that is delivered to the lungs will have a lower partial pressure of oxygen. This drives the diffusion gradient that allows oxygen to enter the blood from the air (Fig. 19.6).

In the case of room air, oxygen is able to enter the blood and the alveoli are kept open due to the nitrogen present. However, as the FiO$_2$ increases to 100%, then all of the oxygen that enters the alveoli diffuses into the blood and there is nothing to keep the alveoli open. This leads to atelectasis and furthers damage (Fig. 19.7).

This is also combined with diminishing returns from escalating amounts of oxygen. Recall that as shunt fraction increases, the amount of oxygen administered does not improve the overall oxygenation of the blood.

As a general rule, try to keep the FiO$_2$ as low as possible, with the caveat that you may be limited by hypoxia. Hypoxia may sometimes have to be tolerated. Maintaining FiO$_2$ less than 60% allows for some nitrogen and can promote lung improvement and recruitment.

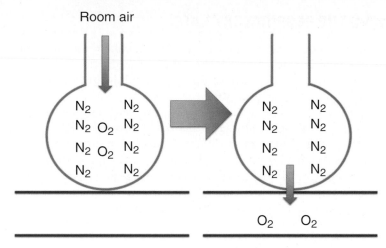

FIG. 19.6 The role of N_2 in maintaining open alveoli in room air

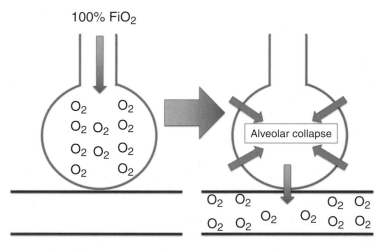

FIG. 19.7 Alveolar collapse from 100% FiO_2

A NOTE ON HYPOXIA ON ECMO

If you walk by the bedside of a patient on ECMO, you may notice an oxygen saturation in the 80 s, 70 s, or lower. The reason for this may be that lung-protective ventilation is being maintained, and high levels of FiO_2 and aggressive maneuvers to force recruitment have been deemed harmful or, at the very least, less likely to be of benefit.

This is an important distinction – hypoxia on ECMO is not *targeted* but sometimes is *tolerated*, when the alternative involves a strategy that may be harmful to the patient. If the patient is not showing adverse effects of decreased DO_2 (for example, lactic acidosis, decreased urine output, or decreased mental status), the benefits of lung protection may outweigh the risks of hypoxia.

CONTROLLING THE RESPIRATORY RATE

Respiratory rate is the second determinant of minute ventilation along with tidal volume. Since tidal volume is much more closely associated with adverse outcomes, improvement in minute ventilation/CO_2 clearance is usually accomplished through increases in respiratory rate in patients not supported by ECMO.

However, at a certain point, respiratory rate can be so high as to minimize the effectiveness. At rates greater than 30–34, there is limited chest recoil between breaths, and a higher proportion of the breath that is only moving through anatomic dead space, such as the trachea and bronchi. Think of a dog that is panting – high respiratory rate, but a very limited exchange of gases.

Now consider the patient on ECMO. This patient is much less dependent on minute ventilation for CO_2 clearance. Decreasing the respiratory rate has several positive effects to include:

1. Better chest recoil and ventilation with the breaths delivered
2. Less chance of incomplete exhalation leading to auto-PEEP, with potential hemodynamic consequences
3. Less overall strain on the respiratory apparatus

You want to allow enough of a rate to keep the patient comfortable, and to allow for some exchange of gas throughout the lung. In general, the accepted number is somewhere between **8 and 20 breaths per minute**.

Be warned, however, that respiratory rate may be very difficult to actually control, no matter what is set to the ventilator. This is because there may exist an impetus to breathe quickly despite the $PaCO_2$ and PaO_2 levels that the patient is experiencing.

The drive to breathe is a complex process that is driven by multiple pathways and receptors throughout the central nervous system to include central chemoreceptors located in the medulla that drive respiratory rate based on CO_2/O_2 levels in the blood, the pneumotaxic center in the pons that drives normal respiratory drive, and irritant/J receptors that exist at the level of the lungs. As part of our primitive reflexes, these irritant/J receptors can stimulate fast breathing in the setting of lung inflammation, as is common in patients with lung/heart failure.

The take-home point being that patients may breathe fast as a function of their underlying disease process. This high respiratory rate may be tolerated or mitigated through higher sedation, weighing the relative risks and benefits.

EXTUBATION ON ECMO: WHY USE THE VENTILATOR AT ALL?

It is now four days later for our patient that we met at the beginning of this chapter. We have decreased driving pressure and tidal volumes in such a manner to allow for ultra–lung-protective ventilation. FiO_2 is now down to 40%. PEEP has been optimized and remains at 8. Respiratory rate was taken down to a reasonable range of 16 before transitioning the patient to spontaneous mode, which he is tolerating well.

Should we continue weaning? Do we need the ventilator at all?

Extubating and taking the patient off the ventilator is an intriguing possibility. The best way to avoid complications such as ventilator-associated pneumonia and ventilator-induced lung injury is to take the ventilator out of the room!

Normally, ventilator-weaning parameters are well established in an ICU to facilitate timely cessation of mechanical ventilation, with the intended consequence of decreasing ventilator times and length of stay. These parameters should be considered for patients on ECMO but should be contextualized – the severity and pathology of cardiac/respiratory failure should be considered as well as the fact that the ECMO circuit may make some parameters such as $PaCO_2$ and PaO_2 look falsely reassuring. Prior to consideration of extubation on ECMO, the following three conditions must be met.

Condition For Extubation #1: Ventilator Is Not Needed to Maintain Respiratory Parameters

"Why do we even need the ventilator on ECMO? Isn't the circuit was providing for ventilation/oxygenation?" you may be asking yourself.

Recall our discussion on the limits of the membrane oxygenator in Chapter 10 and our illustration of the tennis court. We mentioned how the surface area for gas exchange is almost 40 times larger for the lungs and 1/10 the thickness. This means that even if lungs are severely compromised, they may be needed to maintain oxygenation/ventilation while on ECMO.

The main change that will be lost during extubation will be the loss of PEEP. This PEEP may lead to significant derecruitment and loss of oxygenation on the part of the native lungs. Whenever possible, efforts to provide safe, lung-protective recruitment (intermittent positive pressure ventilation, respiratory treatments, incentive spirometry, use of tracheal speaking valve, upright/seated positioning, and even noninvasive positive pressure ventilation in some cases) should be considered for patients who are extubated, especially right after extubation.

Condition For Extubation #2: Ventilator Is Not Needed to Maintain Hemodynamic Parameters

PEEP increases the overall intrathoracic pressure, which can impact hemodynamics and the overall function of the heart. In some cases, PEEP can worsen the function of the heart, where in other cases PEEP can improve cardiac function.

In either case, the hemodynamic effects of the loss of PEEP should be considered prior to proceeding to extubation.

Condition For Extubation #3: Ventilator Is Not Needed to Maintain Airway

Besides optimization of oxygenation/ventilation, the other main advantage of the ventilator is the protection of the airway either due to loss of mental status or excessive risk of aspiration. Loss of mental status is a way that the clinical presentation of patients on ECMO can be deceiving. Because the circuit is providing oxygenation and ventilation, patients may breathe comfortably, with no signs of distress. However, this does not mean that they will be able to robustly protect their airway when the endotracheal tube is removed. This places the patient at risk for aspiration, which can be disastrous in the setting of an already present cardiac/respiratory failure.

Going along with this concept is ensuring protection from anything that could be aspirated. Considerations here include heavy oral/respiratory secretions, vomiting/high gastric output, or blood (hematemesis, epistaxis, hemoptysis).

Finally, when considering airway protection, consider the anticipated clinical course. For example, if trips to the OR/catheterization lab are anticipated, mental status has been waxing/waning due, or evolving infiltrates on the chest X-ray indicate that respiratory function may be worsening, then leaving the endotracheal tube in place may be prudent in the near term.

If all conditions are met, extubation has many advantages to include reduced sedation requirements, decreased delirium, facilitation of rehabilitation, and an improved ability for the patient to communicate with family and loved ones.

PUTTING IT TOGETHER

We discussed the principles behind the settings commonly seen in ECMO. To review, the following are the goals that we can attempt to meet during mechanical ventilation.

> **Goals during mechanical ventilation**
> Spontaneous mode when clinically tolerated
> FiO_2 as low as possible (ideally <60%)
> PEEP: 8–12 cm H_2O
> Tidal volume in controlled mode: <4 mL/kg
> Driving pressure in controlled mode: <15 cm H_2O
> Respiratory rate: 8–20 breaths/min
> Extubation when not limited by hemodynamics, airway protection, or derecruitment

The mechanical ventilation strategy on ECMO is complex and can take a lifetime to master. Rather than providing a comprehensive approach to mechanical ventilation, this chapter aims to help give reasoning and principles behind the mechanical ventilation settings most commonly used while supporting patients on ECMO, both due to cardiac and respiratory failure.

Hopefully, the discussion can be a starting point to introduce concepts, with the understanding that individual patients will have unique needs that will dictate the ideal strategy. If your strategy is allowing for minimal damage from the ventilator and facilitating heart/lung recovery, then this is a good indicator that you are heading the right direction.

SUGGESTED READING

Acute Respiratory Distress Syndrome Network. (2000). Ventilation with lower tidal volumes as compared with traditional tidal volumes for acute lung injury and the acute respiratory distress syndrome 342.18. New England Journal of Medicine, 1301–1308.

Amato, M. (2015). Driving pressure and survival in the acute respiratory distress syndrome. New England Journal of Medicine, 747–755.

Crotti, S., Bottino, N., & Spinelli, E. (2018). Spontaneous breathing during veno-venous extracorporeal membrane oxygenation. *Journal of Thoracic Disease, 10*(Suppl 5), S661.

Marhong, J. D., Telesnicki, T., Munshi, L., Del Sorbo, L., Detsky, M., & Fan, E. (2014). Mechanical ventilation during extracorporeal membrane oxygenation. An international survey. *Annals of the American Thoracic Society, 11*(6), 956–961.

Schmidt, M., Pham, T., Arcadipane, A., Agerstrand, C., Ohshimo, S., & Pellegrino, V., et al. (2019). Mechanical ventilation management during ECMO for ARDS: an international multicenter prospective cohort. *American Journal of Respiratory and Critical Care Medicine, 200*(8), 1002–1012.

20

Anticoagulation and Bleeding Management

When I am consenting a family for extracorporeal membrane oxygenation (ECMO) and discussing the risks and benefits to initiating support, bleeding and clotting are the most common risks that are brought up, second only to the procedure itself. When we consider ECMO for patients, we are weighing the benefits against the risks, chief of which are bleeding and thrombosis.

This is not surprising. Bleeding is the most common complication reported in ECMO, occurring in as many as half of all cases, with clotting/thrombosis not far behind, occurring in a quarter to a third of all cases. While bleeding/thrombosis are common, we can equip ourselves with a much better ability to manage and mitigate these complications by developing an understanding of the mechanisms by which we are able to anticoagulate the blood and how those lead to bleeding in patients on ECMO.

WHY DO WE NEED TO ANTICOAGULATE IN ECMO?

Normally, blood is pumped from the heart, through a continuous network of blood vessels all comprised of tissue that the body and immune system recognizes. So what happens when blood is pumped through the ECMO circuit? Consider the differences:
- It is sucked through a negative venous drainage cannula.
- It takes large and small turns introducing turbulence.
- It is exposed to a motor turning at 1500–10,000 revolutions per minute with shear stress.
- It is exposed to a host of plastics and other foreign substances, which activate the immune and complement systems.
- It is cooled when it goes out of the body and rewarmed by the water from the heater cooler.

The take-home point being that there is nothing natural or normal about extracorporeal blood flow. The result is that the blood flowing from the extracorporeal circuit has a higher likelihood of being inflamed and is more likely to clot. Hopefully as the technology for circuits/pumps continues to improve, this trauma and inflammatory activation of blood will be minimized. However, in the interim, the solution is management of the thrombosis effect through anticoagulation.

UNDERSTANDING THE PRINCIPLES BEHIND HEMOSTASIS

Many practitioners struggle with anticoagulation and bleeding management with good reason – the way the body forms and breaks down clot is a dynamic and complex system. That said, there are some principles that we can establish which hopefully will give a framework for approaching the management of anticoagulation on ECMO. The best way to build this framework is to start by examining how bleeding is stopped by the body on a basic level. Let's review.

Let's say you are preparing dinner – and tonight is kebab night! However, as you are slicing the peppers, your mind drifts and you accidentally cut your finger. As you rush to hold pressure, your mind again drifts to imagining how your body can stop this bleeding.

Bleeding is occurring in this case due to the disruption in the integrity of the blood vessel due to a brutally sharp kitchen knife (Fig. 20.1).

Blood vessel

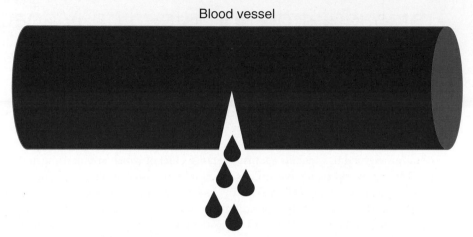

FIG. 20.1 Bleeding due to disruption of the blood vessel

At a basic level, your body is able to stop the bleeding through two mechanisms: creation of an initial web/scaffolding (fibrin) and adherence of cells to plug the hole (platelets). Clearly, both elements are necessary – without the web, the platelets would have nothing to adhere to, and without the platelets, there would be no integrity to whatever initial scaffolding is laid down (Fig. 20.2).

Blood vessel

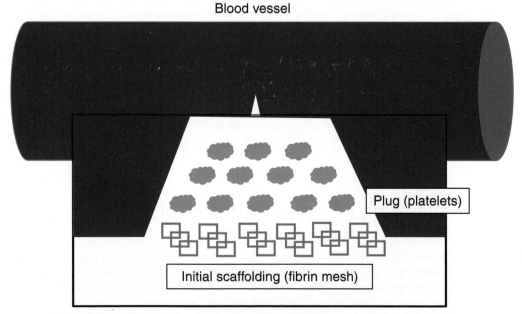

FIG. 20.2 Clotting at the source of bleeding with fibrin mesh and platelet plug

The clot then can become stronger as it progresses from three phases:

1. **Initiation:** Initial mesh generation at the site of injury
2. **Propagation:** Platelet adhesion to the fibrin mesh, activation of factors needed to solidify fibrin mesh
3. **Amplification:** Platelets aggregating to each other with fibrin mesh maturation

You can quickly imagine why this requires a dynamic process – you need to form clot when there is bleeding and not form clot when there is no bleeding. Any breakdown in the system can lead to excessive thrombosis or excessive bleeding. The body is able to regulate this through the coagulation cascade.

THE COAGULATION CASCADE: HOW CLOTTING IS REGULATED

There are many factors that go into the coagulation cascade, so let's break things down into smaller steps. Ideally, you want to accomplish the following steps:

Step 1: Form clot where there is bleeding
Step 2: Lay down initial framework for clot
Step 3: Activate platelets to form the plug
Step 4: Form enough clot to stop bleeding
Step 5: Stop clotting when bleeding stops
Step 6: Break down clot

Let's break down each step and the factors that go into each.

Step 1: Form Clot Where There Is Bleeding

You need the initiation of this cascade to be specific to the spot where there is bleeding. Otherwise, clotting can occur anywhere, and would not focus on places where the integrity of the blood vessel has been disrupted, like our unfortunate lacerated finger, for example.

The way this happens is that the blood vessel that is damaged releases tissue factor. This combines and activates factor VII. You may recognize activated factor VII, as this is what is sometimes administered in severely bleeding patients. This is one of the reasons it is administered – it is the initial entrance point into the coagulation cascade (Fig. 20.3).

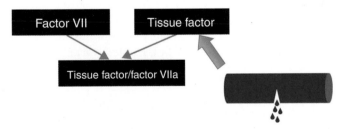

FIG. 20.3 Initial activation of the coagulation cascade through the release of tissue factor

Step 2: Lay Down Initial Framework for Clot

Remember that the scaffolding of our clot is fibrin mesh – it is what the platelets adhere to. The cascade that activates fibrin and allows for this fibrin mesh generation is initiated by the activated factor VII/tissue factor complex. This does not happen directly but rather happens through the activation of other factors: **tissue factor/factor VIIa** activates **factor X**, which activates **thrombin**, which activates **fibrinogen** (Fig. 20.4).

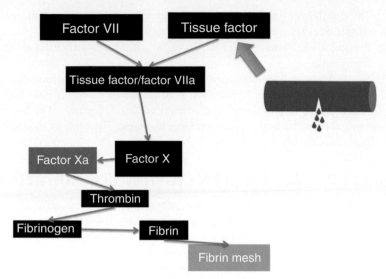

FIG. 20.4 Activation of the initial framework for the clot

Why all these steps? Every extra step represents a point where the cascade can be regulated, which is a good thing. An unregulated system ultimately leads to a disorder of bleeding or clotting. Rather, this becomes a delicately arranged symphony, allowing for the perfect balance. Pay attention to the factors mentioned; they are not arbitrary and will ultimately play a specific role in how we manage our patients.

Step 3: Activate Platelets to Form the Plug

Now that we are done with step 2, we have our scaffolding started and are ready to start to form the plug! Remember, our plug is made of platelets.

Platelets need to be activated by our cascade so that they are ready to adhere to the fibrin mesh only when there is bleeding. Ideally, the factor that activates these platelets would be downstream of the cascade, capturing the feedback of the entire cascade, without being the end product of the cascade. That is exactly what happens with thrombin, our second to last factor that activates platelets! Pay attention to thrombin, this is not the last time it will play a role in our clotting cascade (Fig. 20.5).

Step 4: Form Enough Clot to Stop Bleeding

Now we have our scaffolding (fibrin mesh) set up at the site of bleeding and have started to plug the hole with platelets. All that is left to do is to ramp up the system, increasing the activation of platelets and the generation of fibrin mesh.

Doing this employs another cascade of factors that is intrinsic to the body, rather than extrinsically activated (by tissue factor), and therefore is designated as the *intrinsic* cascade. The steps of the intrinsic cascade (factor IX activating factor XI, which activates factor X) are less relevant to our discussion but what is important is the factor that activated it. You guessed it – our friend thrombin (Fig. 20.6)!

We should pause here and reflect on how thrombin is the lynch pin of this whole process in many ways – this one factor activates our platelets, contributes to the fibrin mesh generation as the precursor to fibrin, and ramps up the system by activating the intrinsic cascade. We will revisit the essential role of thrombin as it plays a key role the regulation of this cascade.

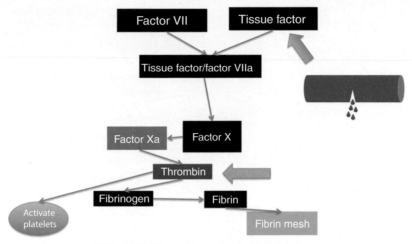

FIG. 20.5 Thrombin activation of platelets

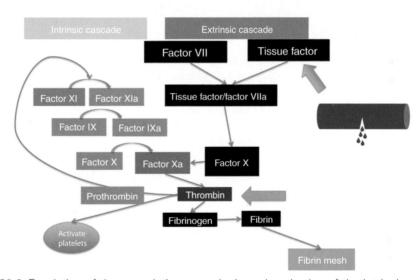

FIG. 20.6 Escalation of the coagulation cascade through activation of the intrinsic pathway

Step 5: Stop Clotting When Bleeding Stops

Congratulations, you now have a strong clot with both activated platelets and a mature fibrin mesh right where you need it, at the site of the injury. You can now release pressure on your bleeding finger and it will not continue bleeding. But the process is not over here. Much like a full bathtub requires that you must turn off the water, the next step is turning off this process. If the system did not have this step, then clotting would continue and excessive thrombosis would ensue (Fig. 20.7).

The system to inhibit clotting is as complex as the system to lay down the clot, with many proteins and enzymes inhibiting factors at different points in the cascade, protein C, protein S, tissue factor pathway inhibitor, and antithrombin to name a few. Subtlety is the name of the game here – multiple enzymes allow for nuance in how the system is broken down.

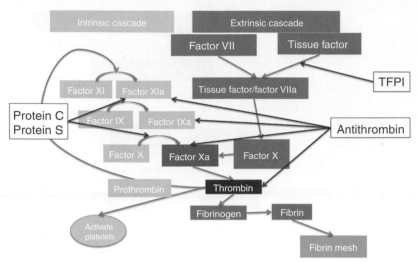

FIG. 20.7 Regulation of the coagulation cascade. TFPI, Tissue factor pathway inhibitor.

Step 6: Break Down Clot

Finally, once the tissue is repaired, there must be a system to actually break down the clot/fibrin mesh. This is different than Step 5 – it is draining the bathtub rather than simply turning the water off, to use our analogy. The process of breaking down our fibrin mesh is referred to as fibrinolysis, and is facilitated by the activation of plasminogen to plasmin, which in turn breaks down the fibrin mesh (Fig. 20.8).

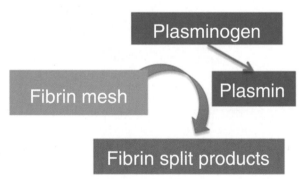

FIG. 20.8 Fibrinolysis through plasminogen activation

ANTICOAGULATION AND ECMO

Even though there was a lot here, we now have a framework that we can apply to better understand the way we use anticoagulation on ECMO. Remember that due to all of the changes described in the beginning of this chapter (turbulence, temperature changes, contact of foreign surfaces, etc.) the coagulation cascade is ramped up. All of the factors that we have described are activated and expressed and the result is that patients are likely to clot. Therefore, we need to employ a method of inhibiting this activation. We do not necessarily want to break up clots, just to stop them from forming.

If we wanted to inhibit one factor that would really disrupt the whole clotting cascade, which one would it be? What about the one factor that is responsible for activating platelets, ramping up the coagulation cascade by activating the intrinsic cascade, and forming the fibrin mesh as a direct precursor to fibrin? That's right – thrombin is our target!

In the majority of cases, thrombin inhibition is accomplished with heparin. As you will recall, the body has a natural mechanism of thrombin inhibition, through employment of the protein antithrombin. Heparin makes use of antithrombin by binding to naturally circulating antithrombin and increasing its effectiveness. Heparin that is bound to antithrombin increases thrombin inhibition 1000-fold (Fig. 20.9).

Heparin is not the only agent that can inhibit thrombin, but since it is the most common, let's explore a little more about how heparin can be used in ECMO.

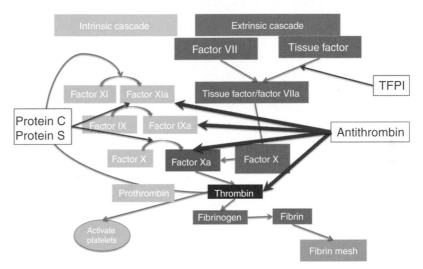

FIG. 20.9 Inhibitory effect of antithrombin. TFPI, Tissue factor pathway inhibitor.

HEPARIN USE IN ECMO

There exists a good deal of variation in how heparin is used in ECMO. We will try to limit our discussion to general concepts, but will give some specifics where helpful. Processes and protocols should be tailored to the needs of individual programs.

There are two ways that heparin can be dosed: **maintenance dose** and **bolus dose** during cannulation. The purpose of the bolus dose is to prevent clots from forming on the wires/cannulas while the cannulation is being completed. It is usually administered after access is completed and before dilation begins. The amount bolused differs but is usually around 50–100 units/kg. Whenever possible, address baseline abnormalities in clotting ability (such as thrombocytopenia, low international normalized ratio [INR], etc.) beforehand so as not to predispose to bleeding during/after cannulation.

Maintenance dose is used to allow for a baseline level of anticoagulation, with the rationale of preventing clots in the circuit, maintain the oxygenator, and prevent clots from happening in the body such as around the cannula or in the left ventricle. Heparin use as maintenance is usually titrated to effect with the aim of maintaining enough anticoagulation to achieve therapeutic effect, without overshooting and predisposing to hemorrhage.

Since the maintenance dose is initiated after the bolus dose is administered, there may be a period where the effect of the bolus dose is wearing off. It will usually take a couple of hours for coagulation parameters to enter into a therapeutic range, signifying that it is time to initiate heparin.

The amount of heparin required differs between patients and titration patterns vary. One approach is as follows: initiate heparin 2 hours after bolus if coagulation parameters are in therapeutic range and titrate every 6 hours based on labs. We will cover labs for measuring effect of heparin later. Bolus doses of heparin during maintenance dosing can lead to overshooting – the risks and benefits should be considered by the treatment team.

Whenever possible, administer heparin to the circuit, attaching to the pre-membrane port if available.

MEASURING THE EFFECT OF HEPARIN

Like most interventions that we have covered to this point, anticoagulation requires diligent observation of the effect, adjusting as necessary. Let's examine the most common ways that we can measure the anticoagulation effect of heparin.

Activated Clotting Time (ACT)

ACT is a commonly used lab tast, particularly in the catheterization lab/operating room. It activates the clotting cascade by adding particulates and then measures the amount of time to clot. The result is a very quick assessment of how quickly the blood is clotting and the degree to which the coagulation cascade is inhibited. The quick/point-of-care nature of this test makes it very useful during cannulation or when an immediate assessment is needed.

However, there are shortcomings of this test. There may be variation between tests and instruments that are hard to correlate clinically, especially in making decisions about the small titrations that need to be done during maintenance dosing of heparin. Additionally, the test only measures the length of time, not anything specific to the coagulation cascade, making it less reliable for understanding the individual effects.

The take-home point being that ACT is a great test for quick assessment and for higher doses of heparin, when heparin effect is the predominant reason for prolongation of the clotting time. However, at the lower maintenance doses used at the bedside for ECMO, the parameters become less useful and are less likely to be affected by the heparin dose administered.

Partial Thromboplastin Time (PTT)

PTT is one of the two parameters that are often measured to assess the ability of the clotting cascade to form clot, along with prothrombin time (PT). Both measure the time to clot, but with different activators added to measure the relative effect of different factors in the coagulation cascade. For PTT, the activators act on the factors of the common and intrinsic cascades while for PT, the activators act on the common and extrinsic cascade. Since antithrombin (and heparin by extension) inhibits the factors of the intrinsic cascade, PTT will correlate with the effect of heparin. The higher the heparin dose, the more effective the activity of antithrombin, and thus the longer the PTT (Fig. 20.10).

Targets for PTT can differ as can the acceptable range. The narrower the range, the closer the anticipated effect of heparin. However, this can become increasingly difficult to accomplish clinically. In general, local protocols should dictate the ideal range for titrating heparin, such as 40–60 seconds for patients at high risk of bleeding or 60–80 seconds for patients with a higher risk of clotting.

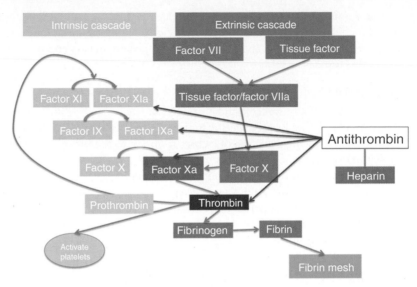

FIG. 20.10 Effect of antithrombin on the factors of the intrinsic pathway

Anti-Xa Levels

A final test often used for measuring the effect of heparin is anti-Xa level. The test involves adding antibodies to factor Xa. Since antithrombin inhibits factor Xa, heparin leads to higher activity of antithrombin, greater inhibition of factor Xa, and higher levels of antibodies to factor Xa. The higher the anti-Xa level, the higher the effect of heparin. Reasonable clinical targets are 0.1–0.3 units/mL for patients at a high risk of bleeding and 0.3–0.7 units/mL for patients with a higher risk of clotting (Fig. 20.11).

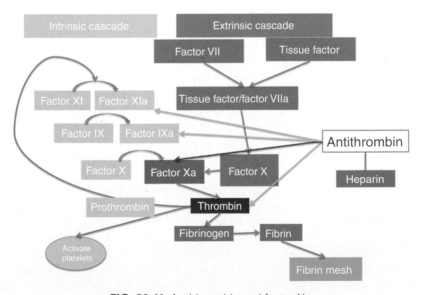

FIG. 20.11 Antithrombin and factor Xa

Since anti-Xa levels are specific to one factor, they tend to be more reliably correlated with heparin effect, rather than other causes of clotting abnormality. However, the availability of the test and speed at which it can be obtained from the lab can vary and may be a limitation to regular use of this test.

Comparing Tests of the Effect of Heparin

If all tests are equally available and cost effective, there can be difficulty reconciling which test to order. While anti-Xa is more specific to the effect of heparin, PTT can be elevated due to a variety of conditions causing depletion of factors common to the intrinsic cascade such as liver disease, disseminated intravascular coagulation, etc.

One strategy can involve intermittently correlating PTT and anti-Xa levels to better understand coagulation status. Anti-Xa will give a more reliable estimate of the effect of heparin, while PTT may be used to ensure that other causes of coagulopathy are not making the anticoagulation effect of heparin dangerously high. As a general rule, the aim should be a consistent and reproducible process with which the whole team is comfortable.

CHALLENGES IN THE USE OF HEPARIN ON ECMO

While there are many advantages to heparin, such as ease of use, familiarity, and cost, there may be challenges associated with its use that should be considered. These include difficulty maintaining a therapeutic window, heparin resistance, and thrombocytopenia. These challenges may lead to consideration of other agents for anticoagulation.

Thrombocytopenia

One of the most common concerns of heparin is the presence of thrombocytopenia, particularly heparin-induced thrombocytopenia, or HIT.

HIT refers to the immune-mediated destruction of platelets that is induced by the presence of heparin. The mechanism of HIT involves the release of platelet factor 4 (PF4), a small, prothrombotic granule that is normally stored in platelets. Many clinical situations common to critically ill patients lead to increases in PF4, such as diabetes, cardiopulmonary bypass, infections, and renal injury to name a few.

These granules then bind to heparin, which can provoke an antibody-mediated process that leads to platelet activation and destruction in the presence of an antibody to this complex (Fig. 20.12).

The simultaneous activation and destruction of platelets in this process is important, as it can predispose to both thrombocytopenia with associated risks of bleeding, as well as inflammation and thrombosis associated with platelet activation.

The diagnosis of HIT involves the presence of high levels of PF4 as well as the presence of an antibody to this complex.

The diagnosis of HIT can be difficult due to the many alternate causes of thrombocytopenia in patients on ECMO such as sepsis, infections, drugs, and sequestration/consumption by the ECMO circuit.

Heparin Resistance

Heparin resistance refers to the phenomenon of diminished effect of heparin due to relative deficiency of antithrombin. Since the effect of heparin is dependent on the presence of preexisting antithrombin, lower levels of circulating antithrombin will translate into less anticoagulation

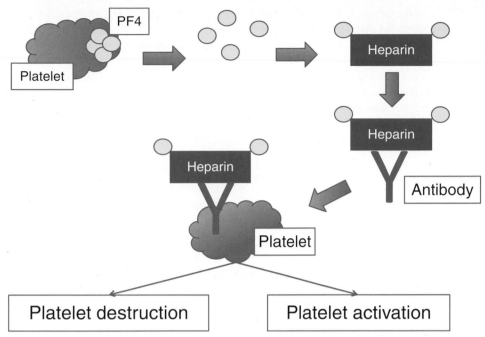

FIG. 20.12 Mechanism of heparin induced thrombocytopenia

activity of heparin. This will manifest itself as escalating doses of heparin with minimal change in PTT.

What can be done if this is the case? Some programs, especially pediatric programs, elect to replete antithrombin. Often however, the answer is simply giving more heparin. This will usually improve the situation, and is a reminder that heparin can be dosed in a weight-based manner – for patients with larger body mass, a high total amount of heparin may be needed to achieve a therapeutic endpoint.

For those patients in whom escalating doses are not affecting coagulation parameters (PTT/anti-Xa levels), where repletion of antithrombin is not feasible or desired, other agents may need to be considered.

Difficulty Maintaining a Therapeutic Window

The final disadvantage of heparin may be difficulty in maintaining a therapeutic window. As heparin's effect is dependent on relative degree of antithrombin, this may translate into variability in PTT/anti-Xa levels. This may be very clinically relevant in patients with a high risk of thrombosis and bleeding, requiring a very narrow therapeutic window to be maintained.

DIRECT THROMBIN INHIBITORS: A POTENTIAL ALTERNATE FOR ANTICOAGULATION?

What can be done in cases of heparin resistance, heparin induced thrombocytopenia, or difficulty maintaining a therapeutic window, where heparin use may be contraindicated or less ideal? This is where some teams turn to direct thrombin inhibitors (DTIs).

Like heparin, DTIs work through inhibition of thrombin activity, which has the effect of decreasing platelet activation, fibrin generation, and activation of the intrinsic cascade. However, unlike heparin, this inhibition occurs directly, with the drug itself inhibiting thrombin rather than depending on antithrombin to do so.

We can imagine the advantages of this approach. There will be less resistance and variability of drug effect based on the relative degree of antithrombin. This may lead to a much smoother titration with less variability. Additionally, if a diagnosis of HIT is made, DTIs may be needed to anticoagulate and prevent the thrombosis associated with HIT without using heparin (Fig. 20.13).

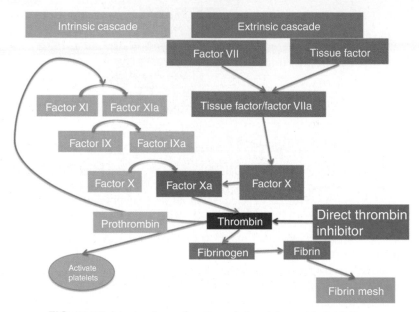

FIG. 20.13 Mechanism of action of direct thrombin inhibitors

However, there are some disadvantages of DTIs that are worth mentioning. The most relavent to many hospitals and programs is cost, as they are significantly more expensive than heparin. Additionally, many practitioners have less experience with DTIs, which may lead to a learning curve when it comes to titration and adjustment. Heparin is still the anticoagulant of choice for cardiopulmonary bypass/catheterization lab, so if repeated trips to the OR/catheterization lab are planned, this may require going back and forth from heparin to DTI, which may lead to error. Finally, unlike heparin, there is no specific reversal agent for DTIs.

DTI Options

There are several DTIs, but the two types that are most commonly used are argartroban and bivalrudin. The primary distinction between them is how they are cleared from the body (Fig. 20.14).

Bivalrudin is primarily cleared renally, while argatroban undergoes hepatic clearance. In general, there are more programs with experience with bivalrudin.

OTHER OPTIONS FOR THROMBOSIS INHIBITION IN ECMO

Remember that at the root, there are two main components of clot – the formation of a thrombin mesh and the aggregation and adherence of a platelet plug. Thus far, we have addressed inhibition of the fibrin mesh and activation of platelets through inhibition of thrombin. However, there may

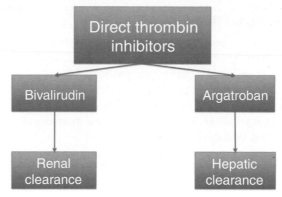

FIG. 20.14 Direct thrombin inhibitors

be the ability for additional mitigation of thrombus formation by addressing the aggregation/adherence of platelets themselves.

This inhibition is often accomplished through the administration of aspirin, a medication with which inhibits the ability of platelets to adhere to the fibrin mesh/vessel wall as well as to aggregate to each other. Addition of aspirin may help to prolong oxygenator life, but should be done with an eye on the additional risks of bleeding that it may add, particularly in patients with low or falling platelet counts.

Let's now turn out attention to bleeding management, and uncover some general principles that we can apply when trying to evaluate the relative risks of clotting and bleeding.

BLEEDING PREVENTION, MITIGATION, AND MANAGEMENT

Why do we have to go into all of this detail? Hopefully at this point, you are starting to develop an appreciation of the system for coagulation and bleeding management. If we incur the risk of ECMO, we need to have a way of addressing and mitigating bleeding and clotting, which can be very common. Thrombosis has been reported to be as high as 25%–30% in the case of clotting, while bleeding has been reported in up to 40%–45% of ECMO cases, with complications ranging from well tolerated to devastating.

Part of mitigating complications on ECMO involves understanding where the patient is on the spectrum between clotting and bleeding (Fig. 20.15).

How can we address and mitigate bleeding for patients on ECMO, especially when the need exists to anticoagulate? As is common to our approach to many problems with ECMO, the answer involves identification of a deficiency, application of a strategy for mitigation, and assessment for response.

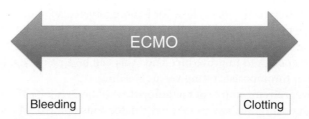

FIG. 20.15 Identifying spectrum of bleeding and thrombosis for patients on ECMO

Identification of Reason for Bleeding

Anticoagulation is a common reason for bleeding but is not the only reason patients bleed while on ECMO. There is consumption of factors and cells by the circuit, both through sequestration by the oxygenator and lysis by the pump, particularly of fibrin and platelets. Critical illness can lead to deficient production of coagulation factors and platelets as well as non-circuit consumption of platelets and factors, such as due to disseminated intravascular coagulation. Finally, turbulence and the effect of the centrifugal pump can cause mechanical disruption of platelet multimers, with an acquired von Willebrand disease effect.

Teasing out this host of causes of bleeding involves careful consideration of the potential causes of bleeding and coagulopathy, with a structured approach for working up bleeding. The typical lab battery can include complete blood count, coagulation factors, fibrinogen, as well as an assessment of the strength of blood clots, such as thromboelastography (TEG). This last test carries the advantage of assessing in real time the ability of the blood to clot and at which point in the clotting cascade the deficiency exists.

Prevention and Mitigation of Bleeding

The most important way to mitigate the risks of bleeding is prevention of clinical situations that may lead to bleeding and prompt intervention when bleeding exists. In general, any unnecessary invasive procedure while on ECMO should be deferred if clinically feasible. As an example, monitoring a small apical pneumothorax may be more prudent than placing a chest tube if the addition of the chest tube will add little to the overall clinical course and will risk massive bleeding. Even procedures considered to be relatively benign such as arterial/venous access, nasogastric tubes, or urinary catheterization can lead to massive hemorrhage and should be deferred to clinicians with adequate experience whenever possible.

Additionally, prompt intervention to bleeding can be prudent and it may allow for abatement of the bleeding before hemorrhage gets out of hand. This can include endoscopy/angiography as needed for GI bleed, return to the OR for surgical site bleeding, and addressing any bleeding around the cannulas with suturing as indicated.

Addressing Bleeding Due to Coagulopathy

Bleeding in the setting of coagulopathy, whether as the result of anticoagulation administered or due to an underlying condition, should prompt assessment of the underlying issue. What follows are several steps that may be addressed to improve the overall ability for forming clot.

1. **Replete products if low:** Sometimes the most prudent intervention is the most apparent. If platelets are low, consider replacing. If PT/INR is elevated, fresh frozen plasma may be of benefit. If fibrinogen is low, cryoprecipitate may help to replete. There is no evidence of the benefits of replacing factors if the levels are not low, and blood product administration carries its own risks and adverse effects.

2. **Guided product repletion based on clot strength:** The advantage of TEG is that it can give assessment of how the blood is clotting which can guide how factors and products can be administered. This may allow for a more targeted approach than just administering all products in the presence of bleeding.

3. **Decrease or hold anticoagulation:** Sometimes just lowering the anticoagulation target or dosage is enough to improve bleeding. This will be a risk-benefit assessment of the potential for further thrombosis/clotting versus bleeding.

4. **Address circuit source of coagulopathy:** If the circuit itself is suspected to be the source of the coagulopathy, due to an older oxygenator consuming of fibrin/platelets, consideration can be

given to changing out the oxygenator. This decision will have to consider risks and benefits of an oxygenator change out.

Consideration can also be given to improving the clot strength while on anticoagulation as detailed later.

IMPROVING CLOT STRENGTH WHILE ON ANTICOAGULATION

As you will recall, Step 6 of our clot regulation process involved breaking down the clot once bleeding subsides. This is accomplished by the activation of plasminogen to plasmin, which breaks down the fibrin mesh into fibrin split products (Fig. 20.16).

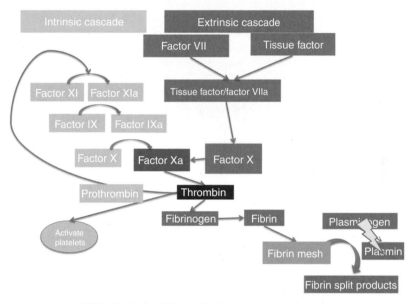

FIG. 20.16 Inhibition of plasminogen activation

Drugs such as transexemic acid and aminocaproic acid inhibit this activation of plasminogen to plasmin. Therefore, the process of fibrinolysis is inhibited. The result is that clots that are already formed are better stabilized and less likely to break down. This strategy can carry the additional advantage of being combined with anticoagulation, with the rationale being that new clots are less likely to form but clots that are formed are less likely to breakdown. This can allow for mitigation of both clotting and bleeding for patients that are at risk for both.

PUTTING IT TOGETHER

Anticoagulation and bleeding management on ECMO can be very challenging. Besides involving very complex systems and pathways in the body, there is unfortunately not a lot of evidence or consensus to guide practice. Indeed, there exists a large variation in how anticoagulation is used, measured, titrated, and held.

It is with an awareness of the paucity of evidence and variation in experience that the concepts in this chapter are presented. Hopefully, the concepts discussed allow for an initial approach to better understand how bleeding and clotting are regulated in the body.

Undoubtedly, more advances are coming in the future – as technology related to the design of the pump, oxygenator, and cannulas continues to improve, this may obviate or even eliminate the need for anticoagulation. In the interim, a systematic approach for evaluating your patient on anticoagulation and intervening when appropriate is likely to serve you well.

SUGGESTED READING

Aubron, C., DePuydt, J., Belon, F., Bailey, M., Schmidt, M., & Sheldrake, J., et al. (2016). Predictive factors of bleeding events in adults undergoing extracorporeal membrane oxygenation. *Annals of Intensive Care*, 6(1), 1–10.

Bembea, M. M., Annich, G., Rycus, P., Oldenburg, G., Berkowitz, I., & Pronovost, P. (2013). Variability in anticoagulation management of patients on extracorporeal membrane oxygenation: an international survey. *Pediatric Critical Care Medicine: A Journal of the Society of Critical Care Medicine and the World Federation of Pediatric Intensive and Critical Care Societies*, 14(2), e77.

Murphy, D. A., Hockings, L. E., Andrews, R. K., Aubron, C., Gardiner, E. E., & Pellegrino, V. A., et al. (2015). Extracorporeal membrane oxygenation—hemostatic complications. *Transfusion Medicine Reviews*, 29(2), 90–101.

Oliver, W. C. Anticoagulation and coagulation management for ECMO. *Seminars in Cardiothoracic and Vascular Anesthesia*. Vol. 13. No. 3. Sage CA: Los Angeles, CA: SAGE.

21

Pharmacokinetics

Next time you are reviewing the chart for your patient, take a look at the medication administration record. Every entry represents a decision – a decision to alter the physiology of your patient, with all the beneficial and adverse consequences that go along with that decision. Medication administration while on extracorporeal membrane oxygenation (ECMO) takes the weight of these decisions to another level, adding the uncertainty of how that medication will interact with the circuit itself.

This chapter will review principles to consider when making the decision to initiate, continue, or remove a medication for a patient on ECMO. First, let's consider a couple of important caveats.

There is a relative paucity of data regarding the pharmacokinetics of drugs for patients on ECMO. How a drug interacts with the circuit, with other drugs, and with the body in the setting of severe critical illness is not completely understood, and the uniqueness of these interactions extends to all patients. Every patient may react to medications differently, and the impact of the circuit on medication effect may differ from patient to patient.

This chapter will try to introduce some basic principles that can be the framework for approaching medication administration for patients on ECMO, and how to assess the effect of these medications.

NORMAL EFFECT OF A DRUG ON THE BODY

Every time we hang an IV medication, initiate a drip, or administer a pill, there are two interactions occurring, how the drug interacts with the body and how the body interacts with the drug. Let's consider the ways the body interacts with the drug, referred to as pharmacokinetics (Fig. 21.1).

1. **Absorption:** how the drug enters the body, determined by route, solubility, and presence of pumps/receptors
2. **Distribution:** how the drug is disseminated to the target cells, determined by volume of distribution and how it is bound

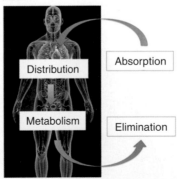

FIG. 21.1 The mechanisms by which the body interacts with a drug. (Modified from Sciencepics/Shutterstock.com.)

3. **Metabolism:** the conversion of drug to enhance removal
4. **Elimination:** the removal of metabolized drug outside the body

These processes allow for a pattern of how much drug is present in the body based on when it is administered. What does this pattern look like? Let's consider what happens when we administer a medication to a patient.

The first thing that happens is an increase in the amount of drug that is available to be distributed. How fast this increase happens is determined by the adsorption and distribution of the drug. Regardless, you can imagine a pattern like this, with a sharp uptick in drug available and an eventual tapering off toward the top of the curve (Fig. 21.2).

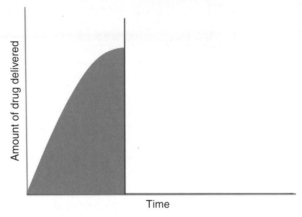

FIG. 21.2 Drug entrance into the body through absorbtion and distribution.

As time goes on, there is less drug available for distribution and more drug begins to be metabolized and eliminated. Initially, this leads to a tapering off of the increase, and then leads to a decrease in drug available, starting slowly at first and then becoming more rapid as time goes on, giving rise to a bell curve shape.

The area under this curve represents the total drug exposure, which leads to the overall effect of the drug. This is important, as it explains the different ways that drugs can achieve their target effect – a drug that is quickly absorbed and slowly eliminated may have a very different overall effect than a drug that is slowly absorbed and quickly eliminated (Fig. 21.3).

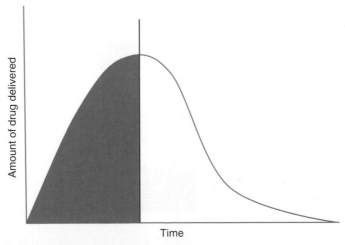

FIG. 21.3 Drug entering the body, reaching a peak level (red line), and eventual removal

How quickly the drug is absorbed and eliminated determines the height of the bell curve, while the distribution and metabolism of the drug impacts the width of the bell curve. Distribution describes how widely the drug is dispersed throughout the body, encompassing two characteristics: volume of distribution (Vd) and binding (Fig. 21.4).

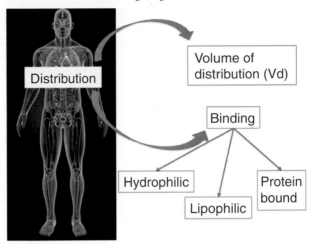

FIG. 21.4 Distribution as a function of volume of distribution and binding. (Modified from Sciencepics/Shutterstock.com.)

Vd describes the relative fraction of drug in the blood versus the extravascular space. Drug that absorbs into the fat, muscle, or interstitium has a much wider volume of distribution, with a consequent broadening effect on the bell curve.

How the drug is bound can be classified as hydrophilic, lipophilic, and protein bound. Hydrophilic drugs have a lower Vd and are more dependent on fluid shifts, while lipophilic drugs generally have the ability to penetrate into tissues with a consequent lower Vd. Protein binding generally restricts Vd as bound drugs are less likely to cross membranes.

However, we must also put this in the context of the amount of drug that is needed to achieve the clinical effect (**minimal effective concentration**) and the amount of drug that can have an adverse effect (**toxic concentration**) (Fig. 21.5).

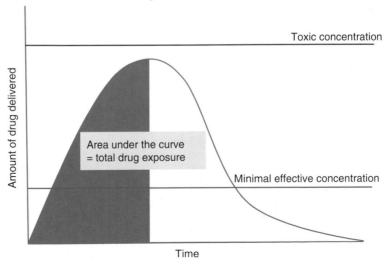

FIG. 21.5 Total drug exposure as a function of minimal effective concentration and toxic concentration.

The key to obtaining maximal therapeutic effectiveness of any drug is to have the maximum area under the curve above the minimal effective concentration while remaining under the toxic concentration as much as possible.

VARIATIONS IN PHARMACOKINETICS: EFFECTS OF CRITICAL ILLNESS

Taken together, this can be a very dynamic process that may differ from patient to patient and even day-to-day based on the clinical circumstances. How can this change? Let's consider just a few ways these processes can be altered by critical illness alone.

Absorption can be decreased in the setting of shock due to decreased gastrointestinal and subcutaneous perfusion. **Distribution** can be altered due to decreased albumin and poor end organ perfusion. **Metabolism** can be altered by reduced hepatic blood flow and altered hepatic enzyme function. **Elimination** of drugs can be altered by acute kidney injury and altered active transport of medications.

The overall effect of critical illness can result in higher or lower drug exposure as illustrated in Fig. 21.6. Consider the effect of a patient in sepsis with septic shock. This patient could have a high cardiac output due to catecholamine surge/vasodilation shock, leaky capillaries due to endotoxin effect, and altered protein binding due to acidosis, all leading to decreased drug exposure.

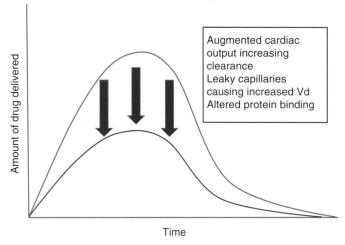

FIG. 21.6 Potential mechanisms for lower drug exposure in critical illness.

On the other hand, the patient may have decreased protein binding due to low albumin, altered metabolism due to hepatic dysfunction, and impaired elimination due to acute kidney injury, all of which could possibly lead to higher than expected drug exposure as illustrated in Fig. 21.7.

To this point, we have hopefully established that pharmacokinetics is a dynamic process that can be impacted by characteristics unique to the drug itself, to the patient, or to the overall state of critical illness. This is not to say that we have no idea what is going to happen when we administer a medication, but rather that the response can be varied. This varied response can impact the therapeutic/toxic effect of the medication, and we should maintain vigilance for monitoring both the therapeutic and toxic effects of these medications.

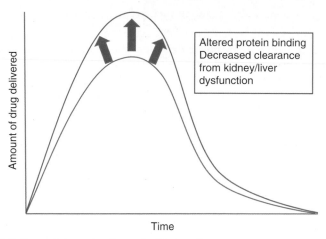

FIG. 21.7 Potential mechanisms for higher drug exposure in critical illness.

CHANGES TO PHARMACOKINETICS DURING ECMO

Let's now take our discussion one step further, considering the changes to how drug is absorbed, distributed, metabolized, and eliminated for patients on ECMO. Besides the effect of critical illness, consider two major differences which must be accounted for in the patient on extracorporeal support: effect of the circuit/tubing and effect of the oxygenator.

1. **Effect of circuit/tubing:** Remember when we initiate ECMO, we connect to a circuit primed with 500–600 mL of crystalloid. This effectively increases the Vd by the priming volume to the original Vd and has the additional effect of fluid shift/hemodilution associated with a 500–600 mL fluid bolus (Fig. 21.8).
2. **Effect of the oxygenator:** The oxygenator is made of plastic tubules and foreign substances that come into contact with blood. Based on the protein binding/lipophilicity/hydrophilicity of the drug, the oxygenator may augment clearance of the drug, or preferentially bind to the drug, sequestering it in the membrane (Fig. 21.8).

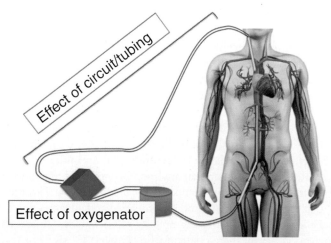

FIG. 21.8 Pharmacokinetics on ECMO: the effect of the circuit/tubing and the effect of the oxygenator. (Modified from SciePro/Shutterstock.com.)

While the effect of augmented Vd is relatively easy to account for, the effect of the oxygenator can be more varied, dependent on the age and function of the oxygenator and other host factors. As a general rule, **hydrophilic drugs** are more likely to be affected by priming/hemodilution, **lipophilic drugs** are more likely to be sequestered by the oxygenator membrane, and **protein bound drugs** lead to greater clearance by circuit.

Although data are scarce for many drugs, there are some principles that we will describe which can hopefully be applied clinically at the bedside.

ECMO AND SEDATION: THE EFFECTS OF PROTEIN BINDING

Clearance of commonly used sedatives is a good example of the role of protein binding and its role in drug clearance by the membrane oxygenator. Most IV sedation/analgesic medications that are commonly used in the ICU such as propofol, dexmedetomidine, fentanyl, lorazepam, and midazolam are highly protein bound, with protein binding occurring in approximately 80%–90% of drug concentration in the blood.

The result is a much steeper bell curve, with a consequent lower area under the curve and less overall drug exposure, as illustrated in Fig. 21.9

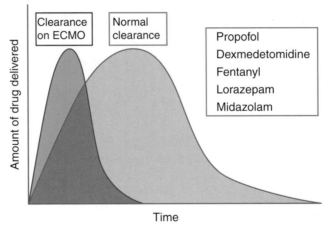

FIG. 21.9 The role of protein binding on increased drug clearance for a patient on ECMO.

Contrast this to morphine and morphine derivatives, such as hydromorphone. These sedative medications by contrast are only 10%–20% protein bound in the blood, leading to a much smaller overall effect of the oxygenator on drug clearance (Fig. 21.10).

What is the clinical result of these differences in protein binding/drug clearance from the oxygenator?

You may observe a pattern as illustrated in Fig. 21.11, which is adapted from a trial where these drugs were administered to a running circuit and the levels were measured over the course of 24 hours. While the relative concentration of morphine remained essentially unchanged, the concentration of midazolam, fentanyl, and propofol fell precipitously.

Does this mean that you should use one medication over another while on ECMO? Not necessarily. Each drug has its own profile of intended and adverse effects and needs to be tailored to the clinical endpoint. Rather, this example is to illustrate the clinical effects of the oxygenator, which may be very different than a patient who is not on ECMO. For teams still wanting to use a drug with high clearance, dose adjustment may be required with careful observation for therapeutic and toxic effects at the higher dosage.

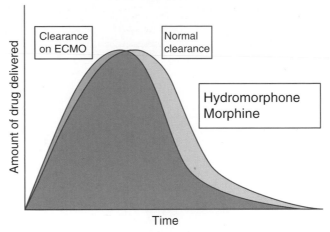

FIG. 21.10 Lower circuit clearance of drugs with lower protein binding.

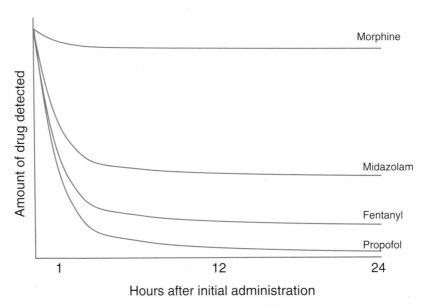

FIG. 21.11 Schematic of drug clearance rates for different sedation medications.

PHARMACOKINETICS OF ANTIBIOTICS ON ECMO

Antibiotics are another example where pharmacokinetics on ECMO can be unpredictable or at the very least, different from patients not on ECMO support. In the case of antibiotics, the therapeutic window can be narrower, with a smaller gap between the minimum effective concentration and the toxic concentration in many cases (Fig. 21.12).

As an example, beta lactams are often hydrophilic, meaning that the higher Vd can decrease the area under the curve that occurs above the minimum effective concentration. The effect of this lower drug exposure may mean less effective activity against pathogens, particularly virulent versions requiring higher concentrations of drug.

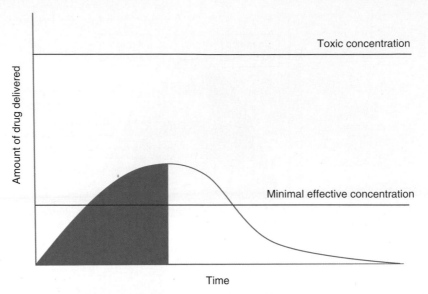

FIG. 21.12 Area under the curve above the minimal effective concentration for antibiotics.

Other drugs may undergo clearance by the oxygenator, similar to the way described for sedation. Although this clearance is not usually as profound as is observed for sedatives, it does exist due to relative differences in protein binding of different antibiotics and should be considered when selecting/dosing antibiotics (Fig. 21.13).

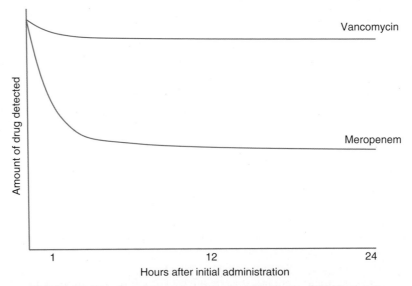

FIG. 21.13 Relative clearance rates of antibiotics by ECMO circuit.

The consequence of these phenomena may mean adjustments to how antibiotics are dosed, timed, or administered. Examples of these adjustments include extended administration time, as illustrated in Fig. 21.14, which increases the area under the curve above the minimum effective concentration while also avoiding toxic concentrations. Other strategies are higher dosing, more frequent dosing, or adding a loading dose.

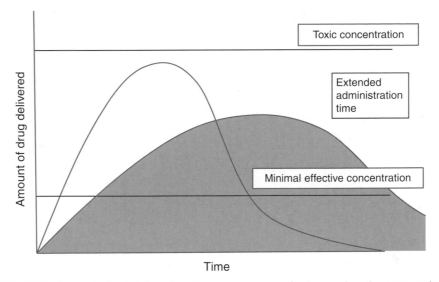

FIG. 21.14 Extended administration time as a strategy for increasing the area under the curve for antibiotic administration.

The other strategy to inform dosage of antibiotics and other medications in the setting of unpredictable pharmacokinetics of ECMO is to measure levels directly. These levels can be correlated to toxic/therapeutic concentrations of the medications, with dose adjustment as needed.

PUTTING IT TOGETHER

Alterations in pharmacokinetics are going to exist – it is simply the nature of the dynamic way that our bodies absorb, distribute, metabolize, and eliminate drugs. Unfortunately, the unpredictability of these pharmacokinetics often increases in ECMO due to the changes associated with critical illness as well as the effect ECMO circuit/oxygenator.

The temptation is to think of the ECMO circuit as a black box and conclude that the true effect cannot be known. However, we can easily identify and should carefully consider the therapeutic and toxic effects of every medication we administer. Whenever possible, measure and monitor drug levels, optimizing therapeutic effect with dosing adjustments as necessary and with the consultation of the pharmacy team. Doing so will help to illustrate the way that these drugs are interacting with the body in the way that is most meaningful to the patient, by maximizing benefit and minimizing harm.

We have advocated for this strategy many times throughout this book, but let's revisit one final time in the context of pharmacokinetics. Effective clinical decision-making should be informed by making a prediction of the intended effect/harm of a medication, observing for that effect, and then adjusting course as needed thereafter. This measured approach can allow for an optimized use of medications every time they are administered to our patients.

SUGGESTED READING

Buck, M. L. (2003). Pharmacokinetic changes during extracorporeal membrane oxygenation. *Clinical Pharmacokinetics, 42*(5), 403–417.

Shekar, K., Fraser, J. F., Smith, M. T., & Roberts, J. A. (2012a). Pharmacokinetic changes in patients receiving extracorporeal membrane oxygenation. *Journal of Critical Care, 27*(6), e741–e749.

Shekar, K., Roberts, J. A., McDonald, C. I., Fisquet, S., Barnett, A. G., Mullany, D. V., et al. (2012b). Sequestration of drugs in the circuit may lead to therapeutic failure during extracorporeal membrane oxygenation. *Critical Care, 16*(5), 1–7.

Wildschut, E. D., Ahsman, M. J., Allegaert, K., Mathot, R. A., & Tibboel, D. (2010). Determinants of drug absorption in different ECMO circuits. *Intensive Care Medicine, 36*(12), 2109–2116.

EPILOGUE: BRINGING MASTERY TO THE BEDSIDE

The most meaningful event of the year to our ECMO program is our annual Survivor's Day. We invite as many of the patients and families who survived their illness requiring ECMO as we can. It is an opportunity to reconnect, to share laughs, tears, memories, and experiences. For those of us who have taken care of these patients, it is occasion to reflect on our successes and celebrate the lives of those lost.

This day is so valuable to me because it is a reminder of the life and humanity of the patient who we are supporting on ECMO. Without exception, every life that we place on ECMO was in severe respiratory or cardiac failure, with a high likelihood of organ failure and death. But this is only half the story. Every life that we place on ECMO is a mother, a father, a son, a daughter, a brother, sister, and a best friend. Their life means more to someone than anything else in the world.

The stories shared during this event stay with me long after the celebration ends. Some are bitter, but most are joyful. There are stories of shared memories with family, of time reclaimed, of discovering a new meaning to life. Commonly, we hear that life post-recovery is lived on a higher plane than ever before, with their illness serving as a reminder to live each day to the fullest.

Rarely if ever do I hear a survivor talking about how sweep and blood flow were titrated, how their ventilator was managed, how anticoagulation was selected, or the timing for deployment of ECMO. In fact, most survivors barely even remember anything about their entire ECMO run. All of the principles that we covered in this book are the furthest things on the minds of our patients and families.

Rather what they care about and what we owe to them is that they get to go home to their families and their lives. This is why mastery is such an important obligation for us to take on. Mastery is not something that comes easy or that can even be fully obtained. It is a continued striving towards perfection, always getting closer but perpetually eluding us. Striving towards mastery is never easy but is no doubt required for us to give the gift of hope to our patients. It will allow for us to have purpose and direction in an otherwise challenging and chaotic course.

I am very grateful for the opportunity to be a small part of your journey towards mastery. In taking the time to develop this skill set, you are continuing to grow in the continued effort to bring hope and life to our patients in their most vulnerable time, ultimately honoring the humanity and value of these lives placed in our care.

INDEX

Page numbers followed by "*f*" indicate figures, "*t*" indicate tables, and "*b*" indicate boxes.

229